The Rape of Hippocrates

A Pathway for the Rebirth of Medicine

Roger C. Dunham, M.D.

Web: Https://RogerCDunham.com

This book is dedicated to the

Patients of America

who struggle against a vast spectrum of

disease

and who battle the forces that are

removing the moral integrity and conscience of

Hippocrates

Table of Contents

THE HIPPOCRATIC OATH

I swear by Apollo the physician, and Asclepius, and Hygieia and Panacea and all the gods and goddesses as my witnesses, that, according to my ability and judgement, I will keep this Oath and this contract:

To hold him who taught me this art equally dear to me as my parents, to be a partner in life with him, and to fulfill his needs when required; to look upon his offspring as equals to my own siblings, and to teach them this art, if they shall wish to learn it, without fee or contract; and that by the set rules, lectures, and every other mode of instruction, I will impart a knowledge of the art to my own sons, and those of my teachers, and to students bound by this contract and having sworn this Oath to the law of medicine, but to no others.

I will use those dietary regimens which will benefit my patients according to my greatest ability and judgement, and I will do no harm or injustice to them.

I will not give a lethal drug to anyone if I am asked, nor will I advise such a plan; and similarly I will not give a woman a pessary to cause an abortion.

In purity and according to divine law will I carry out my life and my art.

I will not use the knife, even upon those suffering from stones, but I will leave this to those who are trained in this craft.

Into whatever homes I go, I will enter them for the benefit of the sick, avoiding any voluntary act of impropriety or corruption, including the seduction of women or men, whether they are free men or slaves.

Whatever I see or hear in the lives of my patients, whether in connection with my professional practice or not, which ought not to be spoken of outside, I will keep secret, as considering all such things to be private.

So long as I maintain this Oath faithfully and without corruption, may it be granted to me to partake of life fully and the practice of my art, gaining the respect of all men for all time. However, should I transgress this Oath and violate it, may the opposite be my fate.

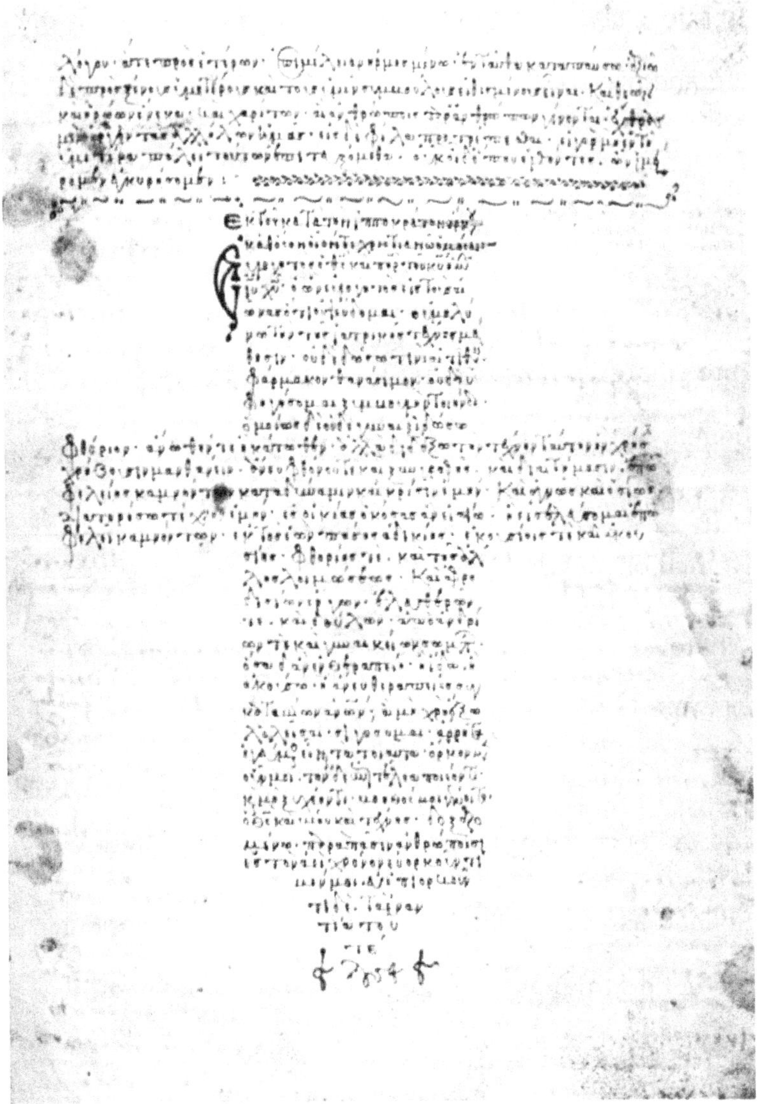

Chapter 1

The Patient

The man was dying and he needed a doctor.

He had made the call to his physician in the California desert community and his wife had made a second call. With each call, the doctor's answering machine gave them the same message: *If you are having an emergency, hang up, call 911 or go to the nearest emergency room. If this is a non-urgent call, please leave a message for the on-call physician and your call will be returned as soon as possible. Your personal doctor will retrieve your message on Monday morning when the office is open. Thank you for calling.*

He was an elderly man, a man who did not trust strangers or the emergency room and so he left a message on the recording machine. Emergency rooms were frightening places where he knew he would be surrounded by strangers, by people he didn't even know. As an 84 year old man, he had viewed the past years of his life, the times he had needed doctors who had helped him through periods of medical challenge. He didn't want to talk with a random "on-call" physician but he would leave a message on the telephone, hoping his doctor, *or somebody* would call back. He wanted his own doctor, the doctor he knew and trusted. He wanted to tell him how he could not breathe, how weak he was becoming, how heavy his chest was feeling. He wanted to tell him the symptoms of his suffering and that he needed an exam, a diagnosis, and medicine or treatment that could help him breathe and keep him alive.

His wife had cried that *she* would drive him to the emergency room but he was stubborn. He waited a respectable period of time then called his doctor again and left another message for help. An hour later, he called one last time and after hearing the recording about hanging up and calling 911 again, he left a third message. He waited some more and, again, there was no return call.

Finally, my father called me.

His breathing filled the phone, he desperately pleaded for me to help him find his doctor, or to find a "good" specialist who could help him return to a normal life. He said again that he was not going to see a stranger in any emergency room where the doctors, or physician's assistants, or doctor's aides, or whatever they call the medics there knew nothing about him.

"Dad!" I hollered into the telephone, interrupting his gasping. "You need to call 911 immediately! Do you want me to call them for you?"

"No!" he hollered back. "They'll just light off their sirens and take me to that sad little building of a hospital and my doctor won't be in that emergency room. There'll be a lot of other people, a lot of assistants there who don't know me and they don't know what they're doing!"

He paused and I could hear his labored breathing. "Can you come and get me?" he finally asked. "You have a good hospital down there...."

"You're over 200 miles away!" I answered. "You don't have time! Please call 911! I will call them for you!"

There was a moment of silence and he finally said, "Roger, you are a doctor and your plane can get here."

"But, Dad, I'm not *your* doctor!"

And then, there was a quick flash of a thought, a maverick kind of a thought inside my head, that settled the issue...*how far would I go and what would I do to save the life of my father*?

There was a roaring rainstorm outside from a weather front moving down the California coast but my airport was a quick 10 minutes away from my home. Feeling trapped into doing what I had to do but I should never do, I raced down the freeway, I filed a flight plan from my car, and I took off into the storming sky. Forty-five minutes later, I touched down on the tiny airport's rain-slickened runway near my father's house. He was hunched over in the family wheelchair outside the chain-link fence next to my mother while she tried to balance an umbrella over their heads. She quickly opened the small gate and rolled the wheelchair across the tarmac toward my plane.

I helped him into the copilot's seat, I plugged high-flow oxygen into a mask around his face, and we were quickly back up in the air. I flew as low as I dared beneath the heavy rain clouds to help maintain his oxygen level, and dodging the hills and the mountains, I pushed the engine to move us at the maximum possible speed. My dad gratefully gasped the oxygen from his mask, both hands wrapped around the front of his face, mumbling something from time to time that I could not hear.

When we finally approached my home airport, the clouds became lower and closer to my altitude, and a fresh outburst of a monsoon-like roar of rain inundated my airplane. I lowered the landing gear and in spite of a transient flaw in the landing gear indicator system, an instant later, all three wheels touched and locked as we raced across the concrete. Speeding across the asphalt with the fastest aircraft taxi of my life, over the pools of gathering water, I accelerated the plane to my car by the hangar. Fifteen minutes later our highly competent hospital staff wheeled him into the intensive care unit where a trusted cardiologist heard the history, examined him, took x-rays and an EKG, gathered lab data, and initiated emergency care for rapidly advancing congestive heart failure.

Over the next 24 hours, with the infusion of intravenous heart enhancing medication and powerful diuretics, more than 20 liters of fluid moved from his lungs and out of his body as his struggling heart became more efficient and his breathing moved back to normal. The next morning, a beautiful clear Sunday, he smiled from his hospital bed and thanked me for helping him although he admitted he couldn't remember very much about the flight. He smiled again and asked if I could fly back up north and pick up Mom.

Also, he asked as his smile turned into a frown, did the doctor in his desert community ever call back or do we *really* need to wait until Monday for his call?

On Monday morning, I called my Dad's doctor's office after it opened, and following a long series of recorded messages about which button to push, including one message about calling 911, a receptionist finally came to the line. I used the "Hello, I'm Doctor Dunham" method to catch her attention, and I asked if I could speak with the doctor, if he has a moment free. She hesitated for a second (clearly, he did not have a moment "free") and then she pulled him out of an examining room, brought him to the line, and we talked about my dad. Respecting the doctor's overloaded schedule, our conversation was brief but enlightening.

The doctor was in his fifty's and working full time, caring for more than 3,000 patients. He had the past weekend off to recuperate from his intense work schedule and to get acquainted with his family again, while the patients in his practice (including my Dad) were being covered by another primary care doctor in the community. *That* doctor was covering those 3,000+ patients, plus an additional 3,000+ patients from his own practice, as well as an additional *third* doctor's 3,000+ patients, as he fulfilled his "one-out-of-three" weekend-on-call schedule for all three practices. Trying to care for the emergency problems being experienced by suffering patients among a cumulative total of nearly 10,000 patients, in combination with the need to make rounds on the multiple hospital patients of all three doctors, was for that on-call doctor, fundamentally, an exercise of ongoing insanity. The telephone messages from my father ranked far down the list from all the other calls that described recent accidents in the rain, crushing chest pains, nurse emergency calls from the hospital, episodes of depressions, bouts of high fevers, and everything else that can happen to people trying to survive the medical challenges in their lives. He had already speculated to my Dad's doctor that he was thinking of moving off into doing something else, somewhere else, *anywhere else* before he completely fragmented apart. The same situation was the case for all three doctors, every three weeks, over and over again.

He apologized for the events of the weekend while expressing sympathy for my father's problems, I thanked him for his efforts, and he moved back to his examining room. I mulled over my own actions, asking myself why I hadn't just called my Dad's 911 system to bring him quick attention. They would have come to his home and they would have saved him. Why should I fly off to get him, especially in such bad weather when our lives would *both* be challenged? I finally decided that my emotional sentiments about my father's life and the associated anger I had felt at the seeming abandonment interfered with more rational thinking. From my own perspective, it all came down to the reality that I was compelled to personally try and save my father's life in the shortest time possible if nobody else he trusted in the medical profession was going to do it. Also, his pleading over the telephone didn't make any alternative considerations seem more favorable.

It had become clear that, from my father's viewpoint as well as my own, the primary care system struggling to provide for the American patient was degrading down to a level that was making it increasingly challenging for patients to obtain decent care. A telephone recorded sham of "care" was being provided, delivering a purportedly "ethical" array of a recording machine's instructions about emergency rooms, unfulfilled promises of return calls, and the scourge of a 911 message that apparently resolved the potential of physician liability. All of it together created an egregious deferment of decent patient care, leading to extreme frustration and delayed treatment that might otherwise allow a return to good health.

The most challenging element for my father, however, was the simple inability to even talk with his doctor, compounded by the absence of any returned calls. With my later reflections, the problem centered on the message for my father from a recording machine instructing him to self-declare an "emergency," if necessary, and to then hang up and go to the emergency room or to make the 911 call. It seemed a remarkable concept: an elderly man given an instruction from a recording machine to call 911 only if he *really* thinks he is having an emergency. That instruction also implies, *don't* call 911 unless you REALLY think you're having an emergency. Furthermore, if you call 911 and the insurance company adjusters later think you were *not really* having "an emergency," in their insurance adjuster opinion, the enormous cost of the emergency ambulance and paramedics would not be covered.

This telephone recorded instruction to patients furthermore always carries an implied liability-protection warning, the kind of snarky little unspoken message that allows attorneys to later say to the grieving family of a patient who doesn't call the emergency system, "the doctor is so sorry that he died, everybody is so sorry he died, but *he was told to call 911*." It is often difficult enough for a *doctor* to determine an "emergency" status on the basis of telephone symptoms and so how is an elderly patient supposed to make that determination? What happens if he only *thinks* he is having an "emergency?" I have had several patients who, throughout their lives, regularly have thought *everything* they experienced was an emergency...they were good people, but they had frequent perceived emergencies.

And, since most elderly people with frightening emerging symptoms often think of their problem as an emergency, should they then *always* call 911 *first* on weekends or at night? Why even bother calling your doctor if you think you're having an emergency?

Furthermore, if the patient is to self-direct to the emergency room, where people are bleeding or there is widespread coughing, where influenza or Covid-19 patients gather, where drug addicts having reactions collect, and where everybody else with every conceivable symptom and contagious disease gathers, is this a good thing? Finally, as an aside, the emergency room is also where clerks spend time gathering "insurance information" for billing purposes, and where potentially enormous charges on the bill are never described, discussed, or available until weeks or months later, when the statement arrives in the mail. And then, the payment for those charges often must come from whatever could be saved from meager Social Security payments.

All of this, centering on the non-availability of a doctor, amounts to the failure of decent primary care for the patient. With this going on, with each patient having specific unique symptoms, where are the doctors in our country, and why aren't more primary care doctors available?

Isn't it fundamental and critical that the primary care physician who *knows* the patient, should be the one who determines the relevance of symptoms based on previous experience with that patient and built on a foundation of a decade or more of training? The patient's own doctor is the individual who can, by training and experience, make the best crucial determination as to whether an emergency room visit is warranted.

Therefore, if the patient is sent to the emergency room by his physician, will the primary care doctor then telephone the physician in the ER to provide critical history, to help the emergency room doctor identify the most appropriate specialist, and will the patient's doctor be available to help interpret the myriad of symptoms from which the patient is suffering? Considering the challenges of an elderly patient suddenly arriving in the emergency room, often a patient who may not be able to adequately communicate, wouldn't the primary care physician's call *in advance* be critically helpful for the care of the patient? Finally, will the primary care doctor actually *show up* in the emergency room to provide comfort and to discuss with the medical team there the correct diagnosis and treatment?

How many patients either call 911 or just drive to the emergency room and find themselves sitting there in a room, waiting and waiting as violence cases, trauma cases, or drug reaction cases are rushed into immediate therapy and care? One recent case in my practice illustrates this problem of an intelligent woman driven by her husband to the emergency room with chest discomfort symptoms who then had her blood studies drawn, her EKG performed, her CXR taken, and then an MRI of her chest taken as she then sat for another hour, waiting, and waiting some more for somebody, *anybody*, to tell her what was going on as her husband sat out in the "waiting room," also waiting for answers. Finally, without any input or word from her trusted primary care doctor, without any input to or from her husband, she is advised she needs to undergo major thoracic (chest) surgery in 30 minutes since the radiologist has determined her "ascending aorta has an aneurism," a big dissection of the artery she is told, a life-threatening aneurism that needs immediate repair. Since the family doctor is nowhere to be found, since there is no information about the quality of the surgeon rushing into the case, since nobody has supplied critical details about her past history, she finally asks in a small voice, could somebody could please tell her husband?

There are many cases, however, when the patient can, by a clear description of symptoms, almost hand the diagnosis over the telephone to his or her own doctor, if the patient understands some of the more important medical elements of the problem. For my father, if he could have talked with his doctor on the telephone, he could have been asked about his current weight (up 20 pounds in the past couple of days) he could have been asked if he had chest pressure or pains (an acute myocardial infarction or a blood clot, either circumstance a 911 mandatory indication). The doctor could have asked if the patient was having swelling of his legs, an indication of right heart failure. Or the doctor could have actually, *actually*, made a house call, prescribed diuretics and perhaps digitalis, and he could have quickly drawn a blood sample (didn't they teach this in medical school, in internship, in medical residency)? Also, there is, *actually* a simple blood test (a "brain natriuretic peptide," a BNP) that costs around $100 and that can accurately indicate the strong probability of congestive heart failure. For the doctor to make a house call…couldn't that actually be done? Is it impossible for a doctor who could come to the patient's home to bring with him a portable EKG machine for a quick 20-second electrocardiogram that can narrow the diagnostic (and treatment) possibilities?

For house calls to be replaced by a recorded message instructing a patient to go the emergency room or call 911, is that good medical care?

This pattern of non-responsiveness of primary care physicians to a patient's distress has increasingly become *emblematic* of medicine and is, in reality, a worsening failure of primary care as well as the diminishment of the essence behind the Hippocratic Oath. Also, this component of our health care system is gradually failing to provide for the expanding population in our country, where the number of patients who need care is ever increasing. Patients would give almost *anything* to have a trusted doctor come to his or her bedside if illness strikes, or at least for the doctor to be readily available on the telephone. A recording that says "another doctor will call" is not helpful when the other doctor not only does not even know the patient, but is so overloaded that he or she cannot call or the call is greatly delayed.

It appears that this worsening problem in American medicine has no end in sight.

While the population of the United States has increased by 21 million people in the past 10 years (from 309 million people to nearly 330 million), the number of primary care doctors has increased by only about 11,000 during that same time (from 209,000 to 220,000) representing a workload of nearly 2,000 *new* available patients for each newly trained doctor.[1] Furthermore, as doctors enter the system and begin the training time that can take a decade or more, while income is near zero, it is obvious that a higher-paying specialty will allow an earlier recovery from crushing debt...so obvious that only 36 per cent of these medical students will eventually be available to provide primary care.[2] And yet, as doctors are retiring ever more quickly, a large number of *available* primary care physicians for our expanding population is declining.

Although the number of medical school graduates has more recently been rising, the stagnation from 1984-2006 in the number of physicians produced each year[3] has created severe consequences. A further worrisome evolution is that, even if a physician becomes available, and an acute care hospital bed is needed, the number of available beds for these patients in the United States continues to drop to one of the lowest levels in the world. The filling of beds in pandemics, as we have recently seen from Covid, makes it even worse. How many beds are available for people in different countries? Japan, for example, has 7.8 beds per 1,000 people and the developed world average is 4.2; the number of available beds in the United States has plummeted to 2.5 beds.[4]

In more populous states like California, the situation is worse, where the patient population in the past 60 years has *doubled*, from about 16 million to almost 34 million,[5] with a large number of additional uncounted undocumented persons, many of them needing healthcare. The current California Governor, Gavin Newsom, recently signed a measure allowing illegal aliens access to the taxpayer-funded Medicaid program, and the state officials expect the plan will cover an additional 90,000 people.[6] During this same period of time, the number of medical schools in California has remained constant, and only 12 universities have Doctor of Medicine programs.[7] If the population of patients doubles, shouldn't the number of available doctors trained by that state increase by a similar amount or should California just keep draining more and more doctors trained in other states while seeking additional foreign-trained physicians?

And so with all of this going on, how does a patient like my father, living in a small desert community, find a good doctor? How does a patient in a larger city find a good doctor? How can a patient *anywhere* find a knowledgeable and sympathetic primary care physician, a man or a woman who will be there to care, to treat, and to cure?

The sources of information about finding physicians are plentiful and yet notoriously unreliable. Decades ago, a patient might turn to the yellow pages for a listing of available primary care physicians in the local community. Now, in our era of connectivity, entering the name of your town or city will reliably produce numerous doctors, often with a "star system" that rates doctors, and publishes comments from happy (or often irritable) patients. Both of these methods are almost useless beyond the identification of a doctor being (possibly) physically present in a community; internet sites often name doctors who have retired years before or have left the community. Perhaps word of mouth from a trusted friend can be a better source of information, much better, although these recommendations will often be on the basis of the doctor's personality or bedside manner, rather than demonstrable expertise with challenging medical diagnoses. Often an even superior source of reference to a quality physician is that of a nurse who is actively practicing his or her profession within a local hospital.

Looking for a good doctor is a complicated process. You might want to know, will the doctor answer his cell phone when you call him or text him, if his direct cell telephone number is even made available for patients (a valuable service that is done with vanishing frequency)? Does the doctor make house calls, and if not, why not? Regularly, it seems to be the same problem of too many patients for each doctor, resulting from not enough doctors per community, creating the doctor-overload syndrome and declining care? In choosing a doctor, it would be good to know where the doctor was trained, at an obscure "University of the Caribbean," or at an accredited school in the United States or a country with high academic standards? If the patient is agnostic, is the doctor of choice intensely religious, where he hands you his card with a Jesus Christ symbol on it and perhaps tries to pray with you when you have challenges, or does the doctor leave religion to the priests, rabbis, and ministers?

Does the doctor have a track record that is worrisome; for example, do the Emergency Room doctors call him "the Candy Man" because of his drug prescription patterns (and patient addictive drug complications), and is there a chance the doctor might have a blood-curdling malpractice record? Has the doctor been sanctioned by any State Medical Board? Did the doctor recently "move in" to the community (after, possibly, another distant community celebrates his departure)? Does anybody anywhere say anything about whether the doctor is "Board Certified," or is Board certification presumed just because of the Board listing that indicates the specialty?

(In 40 years of practicing internal medicine, nobody ever asked for a confirmation of my being Board Certified in internal medicine while nobody seemed to really know if I was one of the "Board Eligible" doctors who had completed residency training but never passed the rigorous and challenging Board examination.) Is the doctor male or female, and with which gender would you feel most comfortable discussing intimate subjects or having the private components of your body examined? What is the doctor's race, and could doctors of a foreign background similar to the patient's own background better relate to social circumstances, home lives, customs, and unique traditions? (Chinese patients in Los Angeles and elsewhere *covet* finding a Chinese physician).[8] The same is true of Japanese patients and virtually all patients of any other distinct culture or background. How old is the doctor, is he or she bright-eyed, eager, with minimal experience and fresh out of residency training or is he struggling to walk into the examining room with the assistance of a 4-legged walker?

It is a complex matter how a patient is to *know* where to find a great doctor. And, the "star" rating system on the Google search engine just doesn't do it.... This problem is, of course, compounded by the fact that doctors available to the serve primary care needs of the burgeoning patient population are fading from the landscape because of inadequate numbers graduating from medical school, or because of early retirement, physician burn-out, disappearances down into a managed care vortex, where some doctors have entirely stopped the practice of medicine because of a raging anger at the perversions of a system that currently forces him or her to practice marginal medicine.

With all that, what is my father to do besides call his son, who is ethically not supposed to diagnose or treat someone with whom he has emotional bonding, where the golden standard of objectivity should be applied?

As the numbers of competent highly trained physicians are declining relative to the expanding population, the probability of a patient finding *any* top-notch primary care doctor becomes progressively remote. And the real tragedy of this is the rapidly disappearing "doctor-patient tradition," a tradition that has evolved over thousands of years, and reinforced by the mandates of the Hippocratic Oath for the benefit of untold numbers of patients. This vanishing tradition has been a treasure that has allowed, in the past, for a crucial sense of doctor-patient trust, providing patients with the ability to confide their darkest secrets, their greatest fears, and to be able to discuss the symptoms emerging from within their bodies. And, as the patient becomes older and develops worrisome symptoms, will the doctor be there to save him or her? This is a bond that, in many ways, exceeds even that between a man and a woman in even the closest of marriages.

And, with the emergence of Hippocrates, the best of this doctor-patient bond became established as an intensely private understanding between two people, as patients faced threats to their lives by the often frightening acts of nature. As infections or other diseases accelerate into this expanding cauldron of suffering and as illness creates an evolving mortality risk, it has been *expected* that the chosen doctor would be there and will use all the tools available to help save whomever was entrusted to his or her expertise. It is a certainty that the doctor's intimate knowledge about anatomy, physiology, pathology, and psychology, combined with the knowledge of the patient's personal history, would exceed anything that can be provided by even the most detailed recorded message.

As critically important as this is, this "doctor-patient relationship" is disappearing into the morass of recording machines and computer-guided visual calls. The time is arriving to bring it back.

And so, if Hippocrates were, somehow, transported from his life in Greece to one of the cities of today, and if he was made aware of the challenges behind finding a primary care physician for his personal needs, what might he say? From the Hippocratic Oath that so many of us in medical school spoke as we accepted the Doctor of Medicine position in society, we said, *In purity and according to divine law will I carry out my life and my art.* To be able to carry out our lives and our art, there must be enough of us to do so...the shortage being fueled by the circumstances outlined above. If these circumstances are evaluated, one at a time, they become manageable and reasonable, and with the combined voices in our democracy, we can mandate a change:

1. How do we train more doctors? Considering the vast supply of intelligent and qualified applicants, it is not too much of a stretch to create more medical schools in each state. It should be a matter of great concern to the collective numbers of patients in Delaware, Alaska, Montana, and Wyoming that there are zero independent medical schools to train new doctors who might otherwise care for the states' collective nearly 3.4 million residents without importing them from elsewhere. These states all have schools or colleges of higher education, the cities and towns have hospitals that may become teaching hospitals, the states collect taxes from the residents that could be allocated for the facilities, and they could mandate that any student graduating from any such school must remain within the state for an adequate number of years to fulfill the training debt to society. *Build more medical schools in each state and create them in the direction that favors the development of primary care physicians.*
2. Provide "stipend" coverage of tuition for medical students who designate themselves as future

primary care doctors, those men and women who are willing to work independently from the hiring mills of collective managed care facilities. These would be the physicians who would like to work *for the patient* rather than for a manager within a "managed care system." This would mean doctors who may be willing to make house calls, doctors who would be available to answer calls from their patients suffering after-hour needs, and doctors who would *actually meet their patients if they needed evaluation in the emergency rooms and who would help care for them in their hospital rooms.*

3. Train the physicians in the "business" of concierge care to minimize the volume of patients within each doctor's practice while minimizing the needs for them to be businessmen and women. The concept of "concierge doctors" is defined as: physicians who offer the availability of their services to patients directly in exchange for a reasonable upfront fee, usually paid monthly or annually. This concept prepays virtually all primary care services (often requiring no further billing or

payments from insurance systems or government agencies). For patients of very low and limited income, government payment of the concierge fee would be vastly less than the current system where masses of bureaucrats analyze every diagnosis, every drug, and every treatment to allow or reject treatments.

Have these considerations been advanced by politicians running for office, by those political candidates who purportedly represent the needs of the population? And, if not, why not? Should it really be so impossible for our representatives to bring forth concrete resolutions to fulfill these relatively simple concepts to dramatically improve the medical care in our country?

And, as citizens in the United States, isn't it time to demand these changes be made *before* we individually might experience the life-threatening kinds of symptoms of my father who must then discover that nobody in the medical profession has the time to care?

Finally, and always, we need to ask, what would Hippocrates say?

Chapter 2

Symptoms and Survival

How powerful is the need to survive? My father made the call to his doctor's office that desperate day, and he made repeated calls, finally calling me, because he wanted to survive.

Survival is the most fundamental instinct in our human makeup, a powerful essence developed over millions of years as we evolved from earlier animal species. It is a harsh and absolute certainty of nature that, without the ability to survive, there can be no furtherance of life for that species. This is true for viruses that might create a Delta or Omicron variant, and it is true for every other biological plant and animal, all the way up to humans. And, if the species always evolving with tiny "survival-of-the-fittest" alterations in its DNA, cannot survive, it will disappear. For the human species, however, it is more complex since while there are not just the attacks from the forces of nature upon our bodies affecting survival, there is, *in response*, an evolving armada of internal and therapeutic weapons employed to curtail or eliminate these threats soon after they appear. The claws and teeth defense used by earlier species against predators have now become our immune system's defense against microbial predators, while medications and curative surgery further allows humans to effectively battle and survive the threats of disease.

Our immune system is essential, and it is regularly relied upon to automatically protect us. Medications, however, and medical treatments to help this system, are complex and must be administered by a physician; therefore, we often need to seek a well-trained doctor to identify which of these options may be appropriate, and to know how to use them. As medical care continues to develop into an ever-increasing complex series of defensive solutions, our need for help from a physician becomes even greater. With all of these forces, and with all of these weapons, it has become crucial for a doctor to be available and to help define the best pathway for survival. And in the world of doctors, for virtually every system in our body that creates symptoms, there is a specialist who knows more than most about why the symptoms and signs are evolving, and most importantly, what can be done to resolve problems that may evolve.

And, how is the specialist chosen by a patient with new symptoms? If there is chest pain, maybe you would need a cardiologist for the heart, you may ask? Or would it be a pulmonologist for the lungs? Perhaps a neurologist, or a surgeon, or maybe an orthopedic physician. Or who? There are specialists for *everything,* and while it is a challenge to know for sure, or to even know if a specialist is needed, it is likely that a competent primary care physician would be able to resolve most problems without a specialist.

That is why the primary care physician has become so critical for survival. This frontline doctor, the *link* between the patient and survival, can differentiate the symptoms to determine *if* a specialist may be needed at all and, if needed, *which* specialist would be the most appropriate one to resolve the problem. This primary care physician, the doctor leading the armada of specialists who have additional years of residency training and experience, may provide the guiding force for a cure and a return to good health. Most importantly, this doctor cannot be a sham of guidance, like a recording machine that blindly orders the distressed patient to hang up and call an emergency set of numbers.

This takes me to a call I received early one morning, at about 3 AM, regarding "an emergency." I woke up, answered the call, and a young woman reported to me about the condition of her father (a physician patient I had been treating for many years and who had been suffering from advancing Lou Gehrig's disease, also known as ALS). She said, "Roger, my dad is in his chair in our living room, looking out the window and I don't think he is doing very well." I asked if he seemed to be in pain and she answered in a small voice, "No, but he doesn't seem to be moving very much anymore." The 3:30 AM house call confirmed he had expired while gazing out the window at the lights of the city after his family had gone to sleep; his wife, his daughter, and I grieved for this good man's loss of remaining life from the vicious progression of the neurological disease. His body was then quietly and respectfully picked up by the local mortuary to be prepared for his sad funeral.

This contrasts with the recording message instructing a patient to determine if this is an emergency and "call 911" where an ambulance would scream a pathway through the night, where the patient would be rushed off to the emergency room filled with all of its turmoil and intensity before the patient would finally be pronounced dead and a mortician would then be called. It may not be thought about often, but the "hang up and call 911" message is of incalculable brutality to those who may, through a 24-hour direct answer by the patient's personal doctor, provide a much more appropriate response.

A primary care internal medicine doctor, a Family Practice physician, or a Pediatrician needs to be a live human being who can actually answer a call from a patient if his office is closed—these doctors are at the leading edge of the healthcare battlefield and they must be available to listen, to examine, and to finally guide the patient in the best direction for further consultation that may also include referral to a specialist. The symptom of "not moving very much" could imply virtually any condition invoking lethargy or sedation, too much alcohol or medication, a transient blackout, or as seen here, the end of life.

And, as the primary care physician now becomes defined as the key to survival, it becomes easier to appreciate the magnitude of anxiety in a patient who has no physician, a patient who wants desperately to survive. This patient, in spite of this fundamental need, is forced to *automatically* be taken to an emergency room or forced to make a hopeless call. As a necessary and added enhancement, this primary care doctor will *know* the patient (important in determining how much relative importance any particular symptom may have), and he or she will be familiar with the thousands of medicines which may resolve the problem.

To make matters even more complex, the profound desire to survive actually creates symptoms that can *themselves* create additional problems for patients. Stress is inherently harmful to the human body, causing a myriad of secondary issues from elevated blood pressure, tremors, cardiac arrhythmias, abdominal cramping pain, or even psychiatric and respiratory issues. This creates more mystery and fear for patients trying to survive as an increasing swirl of symptoms evolve; the efforts required for survival can then become greater and take many forms.

When I was a crew member aboard a nuclear submarine before my years of medical training, we were conducting a series of dangerous activities deep beneath the Pacific Ocean. As major threats to our lives emerged during this time, I witnessed and experienced what happens to young humans under great stress as they seek to survive major impending threats to life. During this time, I learned how motivated people, the men in our crew, handle some of the most extreme threats to survival. During these threatening events, the crew faced the stress from these challenges and created a collective survival for the entire submarine crew, because of training, teamwork, and experience. The patient, however, often is alone, may have no training about his or her symptoms, and often has no experience as unexpected symptoms magnify and accelerate. For these reasons, patients need access to a primary care physician to resolve the problem, often associated with additional symptoms from stress and the fear of disease. As we relied on each other in those submarine days, we *depended* on each other as we took action for our collective survival. For a patient with symptoms that suggest the even remote possibility of mortality, it is a readily available primary care physician who can resolve the emergency. With this physician guidance, the patient may then avoid panic and desperate trips to the emergency room. Also, and importantly, this doctor (like the men we relied upon with our submarine crew) is highly trained. Finally, he or she is closely aligned in a teamwork manner with other physicians and hospital systems, and has necessary experience to provide specific disease considerations relating to the unique symptoms before him or her.

The challenges we all experienced on that submarine, thousands of miles from land, deeply submerged in the Pacific and out of reach from help from any other ships or crew, provided more lessons about survival than anything that can be found in a medical textbook. From the night of sudden flooding into our submerged vessel berthing compartment to the failures of nuclear equipment in my own electronic control area, the desperate need to survive[9] brought us feelings that were really not that much different from my father as he struggled to survive. He desperately wanted to *survive*. There was no doubt in my father's mind, as he felt his own personal cascade of symptoms, that he knew, deep inside, something in his body was threatening his life. In his mid-80s, he knew time was running out for his lifespan but he was not ready for the end without a battle...and so he picked up the telephone.

And, if he had been on a submarine, and suddenly experiencing a similar grave threat to survival, *the Captain answering the message from the men in a flooding compartment would not have told the crewman to hang up and call 911.*

How reasonable is it for a man in his 80s to survive and to expect the enjoyment of more years of a good life, a life of caring for his loving wife, a time of watching his children expand their careers, a time bringing additional days of pure enjoyment on a warm summer day? Is the mid-80s too old to allow this survival? Is survival different for younger people? When we look at our children, we know that survival for them is absolutely mandatory in our minds and in our souls. We are even willing to give our own lives to help them survive. And then, when we watch these young adults fall in love and start their families, survival is again crucial and mandatory. As time continues, as aging carries the young patient into his or her 40s and 50s, threats to survival from diseases begin to emerge more and more frequently and the threats become increasingly deadly. This is when medical decisions become ever more important. The question asking how long can a person live must also be matched by an equally important question, *since survival doesn't go on forever...*how long *should* a person live? Is there a point near the end of a natural lifespan where survival no longer is expected, relevant, or possible?

However, the answers to these questions emerge from a third and most important question, *what is the quality of life* of this survival and what role does quality play when the duration of a lifespan is determined? It seems clear that if the quality of life is abysmal, when the symptoms become painfully overwhelming, the benefit of a normal lifespan may be seriously questioned.

And that brings us to my patient Mr. Bernie Madison, a 47 year-old inventor in the Los Angeles area who found he couldn't breathe as he also gradually began to weaken. He was an intelligent and productive inventor, and he was in the middle of his most recent invention to identify the electrolytes and caloric contents of an apple and other foods, and to demonstrate the calories within. As his invention was finding an early success, his breathing gradually became more labored and he finally decided that the Los Angeles smog was creating challenges that could end his life. More importantly, he felt like he was slowing down, reminding him of the time his car battery was low and the starter motor barely turned over. There was also the distant memory of a grandmother who became greatly weakened and "slowed down" just before dying. Also, with his breathing problem, he felt a pervasive *fatigue* that was increasing and unlike anything in his experience.

As these symptoms increased, he recognized the additional problem that he did not have a doctor available at that time. He had always been healthy throughout his life, and he had regularly put off seeing a doctor as an event for another day, maybe when he gets older. An intelligent man, he thought about his thyroid, something he knew nothing about, reasoning that it had something to do with energy. He thought the thyroid might be like an internal battery that was running down, and he wondered if he should get a thyroid test or maybe somebody should give him thyroid hormone.

He began reviewing the internet for various words to see if he could fit his symptoms into a diagnosis. He looked at foods with thyroid hormone on the internet, he looked at cancer, and he looked at every condition that could cause weakness as he broke out in a sweat with increasing anxiety. Almost everything he studied indicated he likely had any one of many terrible diseases. He mulled going into a walk-in medical clinic, but he had heard they have clusters of assistants, maybe Physician Assistants, maybe Nurse Practitioners, not the real doctors he knew he needed. He considered just presenting himself to the emergency room, telling the clerk that he felt tired, and then he considered the bills that would be forthcoming and the tests that would be done for everybody who felt "tired." He felt reasonably sure they wouldn't even consider this to be an emergency.

His stress increased as he mulled the vast array of diagnoses that could be associated with his symptoms of profound fatigue and shortness of breath.

He thought several times that he might be dying, but as he began sweating from the stress of *that* consideration, he then became aware of a very strong compulsion to survive and complete the development of his next inventions. Without a primary care doctor, which as we have seen is not that unusual, he knew he didn't have time to search for such people; he had heard of waiting times for a new doctor appointment was often weeks away and he felt he may not have that much time before the end arrived. Also, since he had no wife, there was nobody to confide in or to give him advice; he finally decided to take whatever action that would be the most productive.

So he made a fateful and critical decision. He would simply drive away from it all. He climbed into his car and drove a couple of hours up to our coastal community where the air was fresh and where he could, finally, catch his breath away from the smog, and hopefully regain some energy. He thought about eating something that might help his thyroid but he didn't know which foods would be considered thyroid-friendly. After parking his car near the beach, he slowly sat down on the beach park bench and he began watching the waves as he felt the fresh air moving into his lungs and his body.

As he relaxed, he felt his stress evaporating and he waited to begin experiencing a renewal of strength. That was the moment when he abruptly became unconscious, fell off the bench onto the grass, and stopped breathing. Fortunately for Bernie, a passerby happened to be a retired medical doctor out for a morning stroll, who rushed up to the man and began CPR (cardiopulmonary resuscitation) as his wife called the paramedics. Within five minutes, a team of paramedics applied their electrical paddles and shocked Bernie's heart, then they injected intravenous drugs to stimulate his heart muscle, and they finally brought him back into a conscious state. Thirty minutes later, they called me from the local hospital's Emergency Room. "We have a 47 yr/old male with syncope, now awake, all vital signs stable. Would you like to work him up?"

Ten minutes later, I walked in to the hospital emergency room, talked with the ER physician, and found my new patient sitting up and calmly watching television while observing the surrounding activity with interest. His cardiac monitor, attached to a pole at the side of his bed, showed a normal rhythm and his blood pressure was a satisfying 143/72.

"Mr. Madison," I said after we exchanged introductions. "You have had a very difficult morning." Like, you died, almost, flashed through my mind.

"Yes, doctor, it has been, shall I say, difficult...a bit unexpected for me to be here," he answered, his voice hoarse from the paramedic's intubation tube that had recently been withdrawn. "I was just looking to get away from the smog and catch a bit of fresh air."

"You drove up here from Pasadena for some fresh air?"

He smiled. "Well, I thought it was the smog down there, Doc. Just found it harder to breathe. It was hot and smoggy, and I felt like I couldn't get enough air. And when I stood up, I got jangles in my brain."

"Jangles?" I asked politely.

"Yeah, you know, jangles." He waved his index finger around his head. "Lightheaded, spacy, like I'm dizzy but for no good reason."

He asked me if I could do a thyroid test on him along with whatever other tests I could initiate. I assured him that we would include that with his blood work as I gathered as much history as possible. But then, as I was informing him that some cardiac tests and a day or two for observation in the hospital would likely be a good idea, Bernie Madison suddenly, without so much as a whimper or a groan, dropped back on the bed and became unconscious and unresponsive. His eyes rolled up, his breathing slowed, the bedside monitor shrieked its shrill emergency message as his blood pressure dropped and his cardiac rhythm showed a profoundly slowed heart rate that occasionally paused in a complete standstill.

I hollered, "Code Blue!!" and jumped on the bed to begin compressing his large barrel chest while the respiratory therapist rolled in a ventilator to his bedside and quickly installed the intubation tube into his lungs while the machine took over his breathing. As I pumped his chest again to sustain his blood pressure, and 100% oxygen flowed into his lungs, I noticed two things: I could *feel* the moving and cracking of a couple of ribs, which amazingly provoked Bernie to open his eyes and look at me with unrestrained terror. As I vigorously continued to pump his chest, I also noticed that as I created some increased blood pressure, he became conscious, and when I paused, he became unconscious. And so, I kept pumping and at that moment, his heart abruptly returned to a normal rhythm and his blood pressure increased to normal.

I jumped off the bed as Bernie became conscious and glowered at me. I explained what had happened, I told him I didn't think his problems were caused by his thyroid, that he had an electrical problem with his heart, and he looked distressed as he touched the area of skin overlying his broken rib. We quickly wheeled him to the elevator and into the Intensive Care Unit for close monitoring, while a cardiac monitor balanced on his chest letting out a loud "beep" with every heartbeat.

In the middle of all this, the emergency room doctor and I both called a cardiologist for an emergency pacemaker implantation.

Within a few minutes after we arrived on the third floor CCU (coronary care unit), Bernie's heart slowed again and we went through the same thing all over again, including another broken rib and the injection of additional drugs to speed his heart. He abruptly went completely flat line, I injected adrenaline straight into his heart muscle and continued his chest compressions. This time, his heart again came back to life and started beating a bit more quickly, climbing to about 40 beats per minute, barely enough to keep him conscious while the nursing staff put out another frantic call for the on-duty cardiologist to get to the CCU and insert a temporary pacemaker wire through a large vein I had found in his left arm. The cardiologist finally arrived in a rush and five minutes later, a temporary pacemaker at the bedside took over the electrical activity that Bernie's heart could not, maintaining a rate of about 70 with a highly satisfactory blood pressure.

We removed his breathing tube again and he turned his head to glare at me.

"Did you have to break some more of my ribs, Doc?" he asked. "That hurt like hell! I could feel you doing it! I thought I was stressed before, but *now*, I am really getting stressed!"

And that was when we had our long conversation about his earlier symptoms, his fatigue, his breathing, electrical activity in his heart, and survival. Once we eliminated all his overlying fatigue and breathing symptoms that cluttered his entire medical picture, it became clear that all he had was a "sick sinus syndrome" that, often for reasons unknown, created such a slow heartbeat that his lungs gathered fluid and he became profoundly weak.

He finally thanked me profusely then asked me to become his doctor, as I informed him that I already *was* his doctor. He told me he would show me his inventions as they came forth in the time ahead. I took care of him for the remainder of his hospital stay, he never had had a heart attack (therefore he had no damaged heart muscle). His entire problem seemed to be related to a diseased heart rhythm-generating system, resolved by his pacer. His breathing problem seemed to have been caused by some congestive failure from the recurrent persistently slow heart rate, his "jangles" were from his low blood pressure, and with his new perfectly-functioning permanent pacemaker, he went home a few days later.

For years after that, he would regularly drive north for follow-up visits and to show me his latest invention with great pleasure.

Bernie Madison wanted to survive, but he was in his 70s. My father wanted to survive, he was in his 80s. If Bernie was in his 30s would I have done anything differently? If he was in his 90s, would I have done *less*? We actually never gave thought to this question—we would have done the same thing, regardless of his number of years of life. The man lived to invent, he thrived on his inventions, and after his follow-up treadmill testing confirmed a perfectly-functioning heart, he began an effective dietary program and an exercise program. "I got more things to invent, Doc," he would say each time he stopped by. He was driven by his future, and with the exercise and dietary guidance, suddenly deemed more relevant after "dying" three times, he became a healthy man. With his cardiologist, I would track his pacer battery life, bringing him a new and better pacemaker every few years, and with the driving forces in his mind to live a long life, allowing for more inventions, he trimmed his weight and began to look almost athletic as his previous symptoms never returned.

But, without the powerful force of his creative mind and his plans for each future accomplishment, and without physician intervention, I believe Bernie Madison would have died prematurely.

Age, *per se* is only a small (but important) part of the survival question, which is actually two questions: how long does *society* believe an individual should survive, and how much does that *individual* think he or she should survive? Bernie didn't think of himself as being not too old, yet, he just wanted his symptoms to go away, he wanted to survive and to feel better. It is among the most complex questions in our existence, with a huge spectrum of variables. Both Bernie and my father strongly wanted to survive but at the time of their stress, there was no easily available doctor to diagnose and treat. And, while we're looking at age, ask any child how much he or she would like to see the parents, weakened by age but getting along, survive for another year. Or maybe two, or five.... "Yes!" you will hear, with emotional intensity. "I want them to survive!" you will hear. And, what does society think, what do the standards of a community say about such matter? The answers are multiple, complex, and often entirely unsatisfactory.

Meanwhile there is another challenge, in our society. What about a *split* in this survival question, where an individual says one thing about his or her survival and society says something different?

When a man or woman, *of any age*, suffers the symptoms of severe depression, for example, that patient may want desperately to "end it all" while virtually all of society wants that person to survive. If a debilitating disease creates dementia with great suffering and pain, the individual *and* society may want it to end as mercifully quickly as possible. This is one of the primary reasons hospice has emerged with quality care and benevolence in this circumstance.

When one of my patients, a 53 year old man, ordered me to check him out of the hospital the day I had diagnosed the cause of his extreme abdominal pain to be an incurable and metastatic pancreatic cancer, he loudly informed me, *"I have a gun and I will take care of this problem myself!"* Because he "had the answer" to end his unremitting pain and suffering, he declared, he wanted to be discharged *"NOW!"* After asking him if he had thought about his wife and his children with that solution, I pointed out that his firearm "answer" would, in turn, create great suffering for his entire family who would have to clean up the mess after his demise. His depression and his knowledge that he was not going to survive for long was similar to that experienced by an extremely aged person with an evolving fatal disease. And, worst of all, he knew that for the short time left for him, there would be great pain and suffering.

And so I gave him another answer,[10] a potential peaceful and gradual good-bye solution. With that accomplished, he was then able to talk with his family and he gave them his final love and received the same love in return. There was widespread agreement that a peaceful and pain-free ending would be an actual "good" good-bye but also a kind of survival for his family who would then not suffer as much and would not witness or experience a final violent and tortuous end. Across our country, the increasing presence and benevolence of a well-run hospice organization can provide similar support at home or within a protective setting.

And so, what is important? The decisions about survival depend on a vast wealth of circumstances, and what is generally agreeable are the factors that include mental acuity (the suffering end-stage Alzheimer's patient for example), the age of the individual (the younger the person, the less acceptable it often is to not survive), the magnitude of successful treatments available (and the challenges of unsuccessful treatment) for a chronic debilitating disease. They all play a role.

In this same realm of suffering, I came up against a conflicting opinion in a Catholic hospital where religious mandates can play an additional role together with legal mandates, combining together with state licensure legalities. My patient, a Dominic Silverman, was 73 year old man who was suffering from a painful progressive esophageal cancer that had already spread throughout his abdomen when he became my patient and I made the diagnosis. "The pain is killing me, Doc," he said after my most recent test had confirmed the diagnosis; significantly, the pain was more important than the fact that *it was the cancer* that was killing him. He refused to leave the hospital and I kept him in a private hospital room after the diagnostic testing ended, and with his agreement and his elderly and fragile wife's understanding, I slowly increased his intravenous morphine over the next several days to protect him from the painful suffering that had become his continuous progressive reality. In turn, he became, very slowly, drowsy as excellent nursing care kept him clean and free from the complications of prolonged bed rest.

All was fine until the day when one of our hospital's best nurses pulled me aside outside his door and hissed in my ear.

"*I know what you are doing*!" she said intensely, "and I can't be a part of any of this."

"What am I doing?" I asked, looking into her eyes.

"You're trying to *do away* with him, you're not allowing him to survive, *and that's* what you're doing!"

"Actually, no, I am trying to keep him and his family from suffering during the time he has left, I am trying to keep him comfortable."

"But you keep *raising the dose of morphine*," she said accusingly, certain of her medication responsibilities and her knowledge. "He's getting much more morphine than most patients are given when they have pain, it's even having an effect on his respiration and blood pressure."

I spoke softly to her, "As you know, he has been building up a tolerance to the narcotic, and so the dose has to be increased for it to be effective. And, with this patient, I don't think you need to worry about addiction."

She paused for a moment and finally exclaimed, "Doctor! I am NOT worried about addiction! But, you do *euthanasia* for DOGS, not for humans!"

I requested this whole matter be reviewed that day by the Sisters of the Catholic hospital, and by our medical staff executive committee, and I reviewed the policies of the state medical board. Everybody did all of this quickly, and they all looked at the religious mandates as well as the legal elements in our state. It was confirmed by all parties that, for a dying patient, providing pain relief with analgesic medications, or the providing of any treatment or medication to prevent suffering, conformed to the highest standards of medical care, *even though such activity may hasten an ending of the patient's survival.*

The mitigation of this patient's suffering and my efforts that clearly affected his survivability as I blocked his severe pain from his incurable malignant disease were complex processes illustrating how physicians all must struggle to "do the right thing" for our patients. As a primary care doctor, I was not aware of any specialist or any treatment that could have reversed his rapid progressive and painful decline, but I was able to relieve his suffering...to his great relief and to the relief of the family.

That said, we all realized he desperately wanted to survive, he wanted to be free of cancer, he was greatly stressed at the realization that survival was now limited, and that there was nothing he could do to change that reality. He was very unhappy, but there was no underlying internal or so-called "endogenous" depression. At the same time, it was a great relief for him to understand that he would be protected from the severe suffering from his advancing disease, his frail wife would not suffer the torture of that pathway with him, and he would not be in any significant pain for the remaining days of his life. Finally, he recognized his family would move on after him to live as well as possible in the years ahead, and he understood that his religious beliefs would not be compromised as a priest frequently visited his bedside.

The end of his survival became a positive quality in his life.

If this man had been in his 60s, it would be significant to look at what his survival, what his life expectancy, might have been, had the malignancy not intervened. The need for survival has often been linked to life expectancy...almost as if to ask, when you are beyond your life expectancy, are you no longer allowed to survive? Conversely, the term "life expectancy" has often been used to demonstrate how successful modern medicine has been to keep people alive and thriving throughout a longer lifetime. However, the term "Life Expectancy" is seriously misleading even though it may be used repeatedly in much of our literature to suggest advances in medicine.

It is a curiously mistaken belief, for example, that life expectancy will give meaningful information about how long people will live, and how old they will be when they die. Around 2,000 BC, during the Bronze Age, and continuing through to the Iron Age, about 1200 BC, , survival after birth is reported to have been about 26 years.[11] Even very young people, intuitively the healthiest of our population, did not do well with survival. Just getting to the age of 1 used to be an immense challenge throughout most of human existence; as recently as 1900, 30% of all babies did not survive to their first birthday;[12] mortality of these young infants and children has now dropped to about 1%,[13] a remarkable record in light of the immense volume of tragic experiences during the past thousands of years. The overall low survival rate of 26 years also factors in a combination of this previously high infant mortality and deaths in young adulthood from accidents, epidemics, plagues, wars, and childbirth, particularly before modern medicine became widely available.

There obviously was not a large number of deaths back then at the "survival age" of 26; most deaths occurred before the age or 15 or after 35-40. This contrasts with the life expectancy for men by the year 1907, which had climbed to about 46 years according to the National Center for Health Statistics. The rhetorical question for those learning about survival, if 46 years was the average life expectancy in 1907, could it be possible that a large number of people suddenly died *right at* the age of 46, or maybe did they die at 47?[14] However, none of these earlier age deaths was likely, especially considering the fact that George Washington died in 1799 (of laryngitis) at the age of 67. Going back a much greater distance, thousands of years ago, the Greek philosopher Socrates died his hemlock death in 399 B.C. at the ripe age of 70. By 1957, it had risen to 66.7 years, and by 2007, it was 75.5 years. In 2020, life expectancy reached 79 years.[15]

As a result of the Covid pandemic and associated mortality, the life expectancy in the United States actually *fell* by 1.5 years in 2020, the biggest decline since WW II.[16] This reported life expectancy is, of course, the average overall for the population of the country. Sadly, for Blacks and for Hispanics, it is much worse; it is estimated that the reductions for the Black and Latino populations are 3 to 4 times that for Whites.[17] However, apart from the Covid consequences of a (hopefully) transient dip in life expectancy, it would therefore seem that we are all living longer than in earlier times, and it is easy to assume that everybody must be healthier.

This critical issue of longevity is better understood by looking at an entirely different entity called *lifespan*, instead of life expectancy. As amazing as it might seem, the lifespan of an individual has remained almost constant for nearly 2,000 years.[18] By the time a human being makes it through his or her delivery as a newborn, and then makes it through the risks of mortality from childhood diseases, the expected number of years ahead has regularly been about 70 years of age...for thousands of years! This explains the age of George Washington and Socrates at the times of their deaths—while the *life expectancy* was a fraction of their ages, the *lifespan* was around the established number of about 70.

However, the lifespan data is not just for the population of the United States. It has been studied extensively around the world and it has become clear that even in populations of humans removed from advanced medicine (such as Tanzania's Hadza people or Brazil's ancient and remote Indian tribe in the northern Amazon Basin, Xilixana Yanomami), the most likely age of death has been around 70.[19] While the *"absolute maximum"* Lifespan has been almost precisely constant at 120 years during this time, the *average* lifespan was lower because of the higher prevalence of youthful mortality.

And so it should not be surprising that my father (in his mid-80s), who was struggling to stay alive with the expectations of a longer life, was convinced he needed to find a physician who would respond to his call...to keep him alive. My father was the same age as many other people who would easily live another decade or two, a thousand years ago, or today. For my father, survival seemed perfectly reasonable, but with his increasing symptoms, survival without medical intervention was becoming rapidly unlikely.

How long *should* a human being live, if nothing goes wrong? It is a stretch to think anybody should live 120 years since the quality of life during the last fragile 20 years of life is always so markedly different than the first vigorous 20 years. Those last years may be *survival*, but most people do not generally consider that time to be *good living*.

But are humans that much different from other creatures on the planet? What about other mammals, for comparison with humans, how long do they live, largely without medical intervention? The spectrum of mammal lifespan on Earth is remarkably variable. While it is sad that our beloved dogs only live 10-13 years or so,[20] other mammals also live many different number of years compared to us or to our dogs. For example, bears can live up to 30 years, chimpanzees as much as 40 years, horses up to 50 years, dolphins can make it to 60 years and whales can live up to 80 years.[21] A rodent, which is a mammal, often lives only a year or two, but remarkably, bowhead whales (another mammal, living in the Arctic) can actually live up to 200 years[22] and is the longest living mammal on our planet. It might seem, from this example that bigger mammals (taller humans?) might live longer than smaller or shorter people. It turns out that, at least in Japan, shorter men live *longer* than taller men; the shorter guys seem to have a protective form of a "longevity" gene known as FOX03, and they have less risk of cancer.[23] On the other hand, women (but not men) who were taller (above 5 feet 9 inches), had a significantly greater chance of reaching the age of 90 than women who were shorter than 5 feet 3 inches.[24]

And so, for humans, whether they are short or tall, if there are no symptoms suggesting something internally is going wrong, and if the mind is remaining clear, there should be great satisfaction at living 85-90 years...or even a few more.

Are there countries in the world where humans live longer, much, *much* longer? While a baby born in the United States in 2005 is expected to live almost 78 years, it is remarkable that life expectancy in America is actually *behind 41 other countries.*[25] In Okinawa (a Japanese island), people enjoy the highest life expectancy compared to any area in the world...associated with that, Japan is *number 2* in overall survival. Which country gets first place in the world? The tiny country of Andorra, a nation in the Pyrenees squeezed between France and Spain, has a population expected to live an average of 83.5 years.[26] It is not clear why the people in any of these countries enjoy such long life expectancy, and although "Okinawa Diets" had become popular at one time, there seems to be no "Andorra diet" emerging. Wealth of the citizens does not seem to explain longevity, especially since noting that the United States is one of the world's richest countries while Andorra is about 10% poorer, based on GDP (gross domestic product).[27] Of course, obesity, genetic predisposition, poverty, and race can have a marked effect on survival within any country.

However, even considering this increasingly optimistic view of survival, attention becomes focused on the unlucky person who may suddenly suffer a malfunction within their bodies. Something serious, something that might require a physician to examine and diagnose. A cancer, perhaps? An atherosclerotic clogging of a carotid artery? A degenerative neurological disease? Cardiac arrhythmias? A sudden severe headache from a developing abnormality within the brain? Or, will it be any one of thousands of other symptomatic threats that lurk from within during the years of our lives? The question remains to be answered: what symptoms suggest what disease? And, the answer can be elusive...the answer often brings us back to the need for a primary care physician's attention.

For the successful identification of which symptom is associated with what disease, the physician needs to have the critical understanding of this symptom-anatomy-physiology relationship. Furthermore, the doctor must understand what disorder within the body might be associated with which symptoms, especially since some disorder that may be resolved can easily cause the death of the individual. This is the kind of critical understanding a primary care doctor must learn, in the early years of rigorous medical training, to provide meaningful help and appropriate intervention treatment for a patient with symptoms. This attention to symptoms, followed by intervention, obviously can determine the difference between survival and death. This is why my father needed to actually talk with his doctor...he had symptoms, he feared death, and he needed answers and solutions.

At first glance, gaining this kind of knowledge might not seem *that* challenging. A high school student who has completed basic biology and anatomy courses, would seem to have an *intrinsic* understanding of the internal human systems that can create symptoms. A nurse would even have a more detailed understanding based on training and enhanced by experience. A physician's assistant who has completed an additional couple of years training at an accredited PA school, would have considerably more understanding and appreciation for the potential urgency of establishing a diagnosis. Back to the basics, however, even with even a cursory understanding of human anatomy, it is not difficult to understand that, if a lymph node is painful and swelling, there is often an infection upstream of that structure. If there is a pounding in the chest, there is possibly a cardiac irregularity.

And if an older man in a desert community can't breathe, any student of human physiology would easily determine that there must be a problem getting oxygen from his lungs into his body. This, however, may not be enough to be useful, and it is then necessary to determine *why* oxygen can't get into the body, an understanding which then leads to a solution. In my father's case, fluid backing up into the blood vessels of the lungs from a failing heart caused the tiny air sacks in the lungs to fill with that fluid, blocking oxygen and creating his shortness-of-breath. The *symptoms* were from his inability to provide an adequate amount of oxygen for his body, but the *cause* of his symptoms was his heart failure.

Unfortunately, this anatomical understanding as a guide to the meaning of symptoms was not much known before early Greek medicine evolved and before autopsies became standard for physicians to accumulate the knowledge so necessary to fulfill their professional destiny. It is obviously a challenge to look at the outside of a body and know much of anything important about the structures within. And then, "let the dead teach the living"[28] became, slowly, an accepted pathway into a more detailed understanding of human systems, how they may work, how they may interact, and what symptoms might be likely when organs within a patient's body don't work properly.

The earliest medical progress seemed to begin in ancient Alexandria, as early Greek physicians began to perform autopsies during the beginning of the 3rd century BC. At the time of the Roman Empire, Aelius Galen conducted his studies in about 160 A.D., which began to increase the world's understanding of internal physiology. While dissecting monkeys, and later, pigs, (and rarely, expired gladiators), he was the first to recognize the differences between bright arterial blood and dark venous blood.[29] And then it was at Bologna, Italy, where history records the first Western "medico-judicial dissection": that of a certain Italian nobleman, Azzolino Degli, in February, 1302. Azzolino had just eaten a meal when he suddenly bloated up, discolored and collapsed. There was widespread concern that the man had been poisoned and intense pressure was therefore created to determine the cause of his death. A post mortem examination (a completely new process) was thereby allowed; two surgeons and two other physicians determined that the man died from "natural causes" rather than by poison.[30] A couple hundred years later, it is recorded that Michelangelo and Leonardo da Vinci both performed autopsies to improve their understanding of anatomy.[31]

And so the anatomical understanding of the human body has evolved into modern times, where bodies are donated rather than stolen, and where symptoms became recognized to be associated with anatomical malfunctioning organs. For unexplained sudden deaths, an autopsy is essential to establish causality, a process which may evolve into legal action. For a compassionate doctor to understand what causes symptoms, it is essential that he or she know everything possible about systems within the human body—the detailed anatomical autopsy demonstrates this essential relationship, while the remainder of the knowledge would come slowly as physiological teachings began to emerge.

Prior to medical school, while still a premed student, I watched the detailed autopsies of a row of bodies belonging to recently deceased people in the pathology department of a huge nearby county hospital. I watched the investigations in these bodies, while balancing my Grant's Atlas of Human Anatomy in my lap and trying to absorb the anatomical details before me. Later, in my first year in medical school, three other medical students and I spent a great deal of time dissecting every single organ and body part from a thin elderly woman who was kind enough to donate her body to our school for the purpose of anatomical teaching.

Although there was no cause of death identified on any paperwork for this woman, we were determined to find the answer. The search for abnormalities was fruitless until we discovered one of her front incisor teeth was tightly wedged between her vocal cords—the poor woman had asphyxiated when aspirating a tooth that had broken from her mouth. The lessons of anatomy, admittedly from four amateur pathologists (medical students) trying to learn anatomy, were thereby brought to our hands and our scalpels, over and over again as we learned where all parts of the human body existed, we learned what strange causes of death[32] might occur, and as we tried to remember it all.

When the outcome is death, where the brain and heart stop functioning, the *cause* might be something so obscure as a tooth inhaled into the tiny space between vocal cords. We felt great respect and mentally thanked this woman for the donation of her body and the fulfillment of the most honorable concept of allowing the dead to teach the living, especially in her case for demonstrating such an unusual cause of death. Also, it was not lost on us that her final suffocation incident, if followed by a simple Heimlich maneuver,[33] might have saved her life.

And, as I learned, this understanding of anatomy became critical to the understanding of the end of survival and importantly, for the understanding of physiology. Our working as medical students, (once we learned the anatomical systems and every single name of every single anatomical structure), allowed us to move ahead and learn human physiology so we could understand what symptoms from what organs could tell what stories. As a part of this, we learned how one organ system interacted with another, creating a spread of symptoms over a larger area of the body. For example, we learned how the sharp pain in the leg could be caused by the spinal nerves emerging from the lower back, pinched as the patient experiences the symptoms of sciatica.

However, all the physician knowledge in the world does not help much if a patient is not seen and examined. What if a person with symptoms decides not to call anybody? What if there is a deep fear that the emerging symptom might be the *early stage* of some terrible syndrome, a not-uncommon event. In fact, this scenario of ignored symptoms, or a variant of it, happens regularly in everybody and, for most symptoms, we may notice them, we may think about them, we may dismiss them, and then we move on.

Is it possible there is anybody out there without symptoms? Actually, no. *Everybody* has symptoms, messages from the body about something internal, all of the time, every day, every hour. Even at night, even while asleep, there are symptoms we subconsciously monitor—the expanding bladder, the aching of a shoulder slept upon, the sensation of a spider (or some other scary critter) running across the face. We may be asleep (whatever being asleep actually means), but our brains are wide awake throughout the night to our symptoms, and we have trained the arousal-to-awakening events to alert us to symptoms that require action. These are the symptoms advising us to do something, to get up and urinate, to shift position in bed to lighten pressure on a joint, or a quick swipe to the face to end the journey of an arthropod.

When we were babies, we had a large variety of symptoms, and what did we do? We screamed as we hungered for mother's milk, as we wet or dirtied our diapers after feeling pain in the abdomen, or we sometimes created great distress in our mothers who could not figure out why we were crying. Just the one condition of "colic"[34] is emblematic of a variety of baby symptoms usually without clear identification. As we get older, we become familiar with our symptoms calling on the need for some action to keep our bodies happy (while hopefully eliminating the symptom).

But then, in the teenage years, new symptoms arrive...a boy's surprise of his first "wet dream" often coincident with a vivid sexual dream, around the same time as a girl's new abdominal cramping and vaginal bleeding arrives as her first menstrual cycles begin. "What is going on?" young people may ask, privately to themselves, as they hesitate to discuss the matter (especially the cascade of private matters) with their parents or even with their trusted friends. They learn, they study the Web where every symptom known in the human race is discussed (sometimes accurately, sometimes not), and they move on.

The routine body symptoms continue without much attention throughout the 20s, the 30s and then, around the 40s, *new* symptoms begin to arise that are often different and therefore mysterious. The ringing in the ears, the sensations from joints that may cause pain with certain activities, the spasms of muscles, the episodes of anxiety or fatigue, so many of the thousands of potential symptoms create the need for a diagnosis. And so, thoughts of seeing a medical doctor begin to evolve. This process expands, until a point is reached, for patients often reaching their 60s or 70s when they may call their doctor for an explanation and possibly treatment. Maybe, for some patients, calling a doctor for a "routine physical exam" just in case anything should be wrong. Of course, for the doctor, the great burden is identifying conditions that may end survival when there are no symptoms...leading to "routine" mammograms, "routine" electrocardiograms or treadmills, a "routine" colonoscopy, and (in previous years) "routine" chest x-rays, along with routine everything else such as vaccinations, identifying family history factors, and whatever might predict the challenge to survival.

I sit across from the patient and ask, "How are you feeling, anything going on?" and the patient will sometimes stare at me for a few seconds, mulling just how much of the plethora of his or her specific symptoms should be revealed. Almost nobody is inclined to reveal all of his or her symptoms, especially those that are personal and private. In a patient with many symptoms, however, only one or two might need to be revealed. Some of the symptoms may be embarrassing, others worrisome, some are new and many may have been present for a long duration. At some point in life, there are often *hundreds* of symptoms, every day, all day, while awake or asleep, often with no clear identification as to the cause, but usually with the certain inclination from the patient that he or she does not need to burden the doctor with too much information.

There can be so many symptoms but what to tell the doctor?

The answer is not always clear. And, in the back of many patients' minds is the question, at what point in the revelation of symptoms would the doctor become overwhelmed? Or, which symptoms would an array of unnecessary tests need to be performed? Most people sense that no doctor would want a conversation to start with, "Thank you for asking, doctor. I have, at this moment, about 73 symptoms...could we spend a couple of hours discussing them?"

And so, then, there is then a *selective* revelation of symptoms that each patient may think is important. Perhaps symptoms that relate to a background nagging worry about survival. This selective mechanism itself encompasses a huge spectrum, ranging from a so-called hypochondriac who worries about each symptom that comes to mind, to the opposite extreme where (usually a man) will look at me as I ask how he is doing, he will think for a second, and he will finally say, gruffly, "Everything is fine, Doc, no problems," with a quick dismissal wave of his hand. No problem except for his enlarging prostate, perhaps from an early malignancy, is causing his need to urinate more frequently at night. That would be a problem he might want to mention. And then, there is that twinge of pressure in his left shoulder, just a twinge when he works out, a minimal symptom that could point in the direction of a future heart attack. No problem, doc, except for the occasional wheezing as asthma emerges, no problem except for the anxieties and insomnias that emerge that keep me awake nights...suggesting marital conflicts or workplace stresses. The slight weakness of an arm from early multiple sclerosis, the slight new tremor from early Parkinson's disease can join the symptom list for an unfortunate patient. Or, how much worry should a small headache, when there never had been one, possibly emerging from an early glioblastoma brain tumor. The new changes in bowel habits from an early colon malignancy. The skin irregularity on the side of his sunburned nose, the pigmented growth on the leg, the twitching and spasms, the numbness of fingers, the, the, on and on. There is no end to the cascade of symptoms that now are warning of an impending medical disaster. All of these symptoms are, however, included in this endless list of uncertainty, and each of them may mean nothing.

A good doctor, *if the doctor-patient relationship is present and time for a proper office visit allows,* can relieve the anxiety of the unknown while bringing comfort from the evaluation and treatment.

However, the greatest challenge for a physician is a patient who cannot vocalize *any* symptom, such as a patient with advanced schizophrenia who may be virtually mute and yet look distressed. Or the patient in a coma, or who has had a stroke and cannot talk, or who looks continuously troubled for reasons as obscure as the symptoms demonstrated by a newborn baby. Pediatricians deal with this continuously, and they have always had my admiration for the challenge of their work as they identify problems from within a tiny human being who is unable to talk. When there is no conversation, when there is no history, it often becomes exceedingly difficult to establish a diagnosis. It has been estimated[35] that as many as 90% of medical diagnoses are determined by what the patient describes, by the history alone, rather than the physical findings during an examination. The history told by the patient as symptoms surface, is the oldest of diagnostic tools...taking the time for the physician to listen to a comprehensive history is critically important.

Since we are talking about patient *survival*, how important is it for a doctor to listen while a patient speaks, especially when studies[36] have shown that doctors interrupt a patient, on the average, about every 18 seconds? But then, when the patient does talk and does try to describe symptoms, is the doctor listening? Does the doctor have time to listen? For the enhancement of patient survival, the doctor must be able to hear and must not be struggling with the time-crunch of an overloaded schedule, cannot be looking at the computer screen, and must not be distracted from hearing the vital information directly from the symptomatic patient.

One of the challenges of being a doctor relates to the tasks of symptom-perception and symptom-recognition, with the subsequent identification of which symptom should create alarm. During the years of medical school and residency, there is a teaching process that makes emerging physicians aware of the *thousands* of serious medical conditions that are possible in a lifetime, each often with potential symptoms that are unique, or that may overlap, and often not specific to the condition. Our medical school class became filled, in fact, with intensely alert doctors-in-training, each seeking and sensing each symptom *within himself or herself*, and sometimes fearing the worst. Hypochondriasis emerges for countless medical students, exacerbating the stresses of medical school as they work to absorb the vast amounts of information. Over time, fortunately, we became adjusted to the false-positive nature of most of these symptoms that initially seemed to be telling us that we are soon going to die, those alarming symptoms which (mostly) just thankfully go away.

However, we did learn that the element of *fear* itself often magnifies the intensity of each symptom, breeding more fear which led to more intense symptoms, continuously down a tortuous spiral of anxiety. Finally, some of us gave up and resorted to seeing one of the medical school doctors for an examination and hopefully reassurance. Through this time, however, most of us became more sensitized to the magnification effect of fear on patients, especially anxious patients, who are (like most other people) just trying to stay healthy and get along in life. This recognition allows us to screen-out or give less importance to the associated symptoms from anxiety, giving a better chance of establishing the correct diagnosis, and providing the patient with a better chance for survival. In short, by having our own symptoms, we became better at identifying how patients were feeling as they later came to see us with symptoms of their own.

So, from a patient's perspective, when new symptoms arise, when should one call his or her physician (assuming one can be reached), and what is a patient to do if a doctor cannot be reached? What should be done if the doctor's office tells you an appointment can be made "in a couple of weeks," and at what point when should a patient just declare an emergency and descend into the nearest emergency room (after "hanging up")? What should a patient say if he or she is told over the telephone that "the doctor's assistant" can see you sooner, perhaps in a day or two? Not, exactly, the doctor, but the "doctor's assistant." For patients who are old, *really old*, with thousands of symptoms and the increasing knowledge that they may not be alive long, what is he or she to do? This underscores the importance of family, where I have found that a family member (more often a daughter) will sound the alarm and bring the parent in, *somewhere, anywhere,* for an examination by a physician sooner rather than later. And then, the elderly soul may often deny to the doctor that anything is wrong, again with a dismissal wave of the hand, until the relative points out the major symptoms that are alarming.

If there is not a doctor available to take care of the expanding pool of patients, what can be done to resolve the patient's assortment of symptoms?

Since the time for survival on earth is limited for all of us, there will inevitably be progression to a point where a survival for years or decades ahead is no longer the primary issue. Often, this goodbye will come from relatives who have watched a family member suffer from a disease or suffer from some other devastation by nature, and who is progressing down a pathway of decline. In this circumstance, an emerging deplorable quality of life can easily become more important than the issue of survival. Since these patients are invariably already under the care of a physician, there is often no effort needed to find a doctor, and questions of survival are replaced by questions about how to best provide comfort during the time that is left.

Occasionally, I have come across cases where a family will transfer a patient to my care after another physician had continued extensive, unrewarding (and often expensive) treatment for someone who had suffered symptoms from a major stroke, or who developed a similar debilitation from another condition. It was difficult for me to understand how the doctor could be keeping the patient alive, not so much as a human being but more as a biological specimen, perhaps with a treasured past but no viable future. The placement of gastric tubes into the stomachs of people with severe mental conditions who permanently can't eat or swallow, the placement of tracheostomy tubes into the lungs of patients who have had a massive stroke and can never again breathe without mechanical assistance, the restraining of patients with psychiatric diseases who have become violent, or the excessive sedation some agitated patients may receive, are all examples of activities that may create a prolongation of pain and suffering for the patient as well as the family. I would try to help when I could, for patients with such cascades of symptoms and such overwhelming suffering, and I would provide attention to end-of-life issues that often are brought under consideration.

Often, I would call on the services of *hospice* to help the patient at this critical time of life as death is approaching.

The vast majority of Americans (80%)[37] would prefer to be allowed to peacefully die at home, and yet hospice services which may allow a fulfillment of this desire is provided to barely a third of dying patients. This concept of hospice to help alleviate symptoms for patients (with less than six months to live) actually first evolved hundreds of years ago, around the 11th century and, amazingly, hospice services were widespread during the Middle Ages.[38] More recently, in the United States, Dr. Elisabeth Kübler-Ross brought the concept to a widespread public acceptance with her remarkable book written in 1969, On Death And Dying, in which she wrote of her interviews with more than 500 dying patients. She strongly promoted a sentiment that people have a fundamental right to die with dignity outside a hospital, that they have the right to peacefully die at home.

Probably the most salient observation on the benefits of hospice came from a remarkable English physician, Dame Cicely Saunders, who founded the hospice movement in London and dedicated her medical career to the care of dying patients. Widely considered the key founder of modern hospice programs, she said,

"You matter because you are you, and you matter to the end of your life. We will do all we can not only to help you die peacefully, but also to help you live until you die."[39]

The first hospice in the United States was then founded in 1974, in Branford, CT, and in 1986, the Medicare Hospice Benefit law was created by Congress allowing states to include hospice in their Medicaid programs and to make it available to terminally ill nursing home residents as well. Over the following decades, Medicare reimbursement rates increased, and additional funding and legislation for hospice expanded to ever-increasing numbers of people, topping one million by 2004 and by the end of the next year, more than 4,000 hospice systems were available across the United States.[40]

Hospice is fundamentally different from palliative care. While palliative care begins at the time of a diagnosis and at the time treatment starts for an incurable disease, hospice care begins after treatment of the disease is stopped and when it is clear that the person is not going to survive the illness. Hospice requires a few simple rules be followed. When a patient is "signed into hospice," it is agreed that there generally will be no transfer to an acute care hospital, that Medicare will no longer be a part of the hospital financial service, and that there will be the need for substantial relief from pain and other symptoms that frequently may occur near the end of life. Hospice is not "giving up" so much as it is providing for care that focuses on the quality of life rather than focusing on the curing of a disease. Finally, hospice can help the family of a patient with an adverse prognosis by performing vital assistance with such everyday things like shopping and maintaining a hygienic and sanitary home.

And so hospice is for the patients approaching the end of their lives with a spectrum of associated symptoms, the patients who need peace and contentment, where "comfort care" has become mandatory, and where the length of future survival is not an issue. This care, widely considered to be *end of life care*, brings together this remarkable team of hospice workers consisting of a medical doctor, a nurse, a social worker/counsellor, a chaplain, a priest or rabbi, a home health aide, and trained volunteers. Also, and importantly, hospice is attentive to the family of the suffering individual, helping bring solace along with an understanding of the activities that can help the loved patient. I have found the Hospice nurses as close to Godliness as anybody in medicine, where *compassion with medical expertise* is the driving force of care. I have regularly relied on this system for these suffering patients who will not survive for long, the patients who need loving care that overwhelmed families can no longer provide as they experience such sorrow and anguish. And, finally, after the patient's death, a full year of bereavement counseling is available for the family to further smooth the emotional turmoil of such difficult times.

It would seem likely that, if Hippocrates was able to witness the benefits of hospice care , he would recognize and appreciate the fulfillment of his Hippocratic Oath *into whatever homes I go, I will enter them for the benefit of the sick,* and would be satisfied that the strongest and most fundamental ethics of Medicine are fulfilled.

Chapter 3

Traditions

How did the name Hippocrates become so emblematic of the moral code for the ethical delivery of medical care?

Hippocrates, as a name, almost radiates the concept of *medical ethics*—ethics for a doctor's activities with patients and ethics in a doctor's practice of medicine. Although some physicians may argue the point, as humans, doctors are but mere mortals[41], and they are therefore subject to the same compulsions and inclinations as all other humans. The long list of potential unethical or immoral proclivities are headlined by sexual compulsions, monetary acquisitions, and personal comfort. And yet, by the mandates of the Hippocratic Oath, caring for a patient is a unique and golden arena that rises above these forces to help patients who are suffering from the consequences of disease, aging, and injury.

Another most prominent symbol of medicine, at least in the United States, is the caduceus. The figure of two snakes winding around a winged staff is, however, only minimally historically associated with medicine.[42] The symbol actually replacing the caduceus is the more historically valid medical figure, the Rod of Asclepius, a single snake around a rod held by a Greek god known, of course, as Asclepius. However, neither of these symbols carries any of the aura of ethics that emerged in the Greek time of Hippocrates although, as medical symbols, they imply that the principles of morality in the practice of medicine would be carried by whatever person or entity displays either of these Greek medical representations.

How can there be subtle pressures for physicians to disregard the Hippocratic Oath? When I was asked, one day about 20 years ago, to fulfill the insurance certification needs for a beautiful young actress involved in a motion picture filming in our local area, the producer asked me if I would examine her and sign the forms, certifying that she was physically healthy and without significant impairment. "It is needed for our insurance mandate," he explained, and I agreed to perform the service.

I took the woman to her private hotel room and spent twenty minutes behind the locked door examining her. I checked her blood pressure and pulse, I checked her temperature, I listened to her heart and her lungs, I checked her abdominal organs, I looked for edema or circulatory impairment, and I checked her neurological reflexes. Essentially, I gave her a complete physical exam. I performed these activities with the locked mindset of a physician performing a medical service for a patient, and her mannerisms and responses to the examination reflected her trust that I would do exactly that and, throughout the exam, remain 100% a professional and ethical physician. I do not know if she had any awareness of Hippocrates, but as a physician, the standards mandated by our graduating oath were *expected* of me. She trusted me to confirm that she was healthy and that I would, as a doctor, help her move on with her career and the immediate opportunities that awaited her. And, without hesitation, she trusted me alone with her in her hotel room, and I trusted her to accept this exam as I finally delivered her back to the set and signed off the producer's insurance forms. The producer also trusted me, *as a physician*, to perform the examination activity with the highest measure of ethical standards without descending to any human inclinations.

In short, with an activity that is performed in patients' private homes, in a private exam room, in an examination room in the hospital, or even in a hotel room, I fulfilled the mandates of the Hippocratic Oath. From the beginning of a medical career (upon medical school graduation when the oath is recited) to retirement, in my mind, this is a requirement that applies 100% of the time with patients, with *all* patients...there cannot be a bending of these Hippocratic principles, never, not even once. This was, however, 20 years ago, and since that time, the trust from the patient that was so automatic has long since eroded as the avalanche of accusations against deviant physicians (as was identified in the Olympics) and against others with power (as in the motion picture industry), emerging and amplified by the press and throughout social media. What was formerly a strong and nearly automatic element of trust has unfortunately become altered in the public mind.

Much of the public *expects* that deviations from the Hippocratic mandates may occur, to the point, now, where females are in several states of our country are required to *sign a consent form* before a routine pelvic examination or before a Pap smear may be performed.[43] In this form, a "Pelvic Examination" is defined in detail, suggesting the patient would know what the "health care provider's *gloved hand*" is going to examine. The process is often now defined as the examination that will be performed "with an escort." According to the Florida State mandates, the form is then signed by the patient, or by the "healthcare surrogate," or by the parent, and then the relationship of the "surrogate" is further defined. Although no penalties have been proposed (in Florida), the legislative representatives are looking to control all elements of physician behavior by added the following phrase: *Providers should appreciate the potential for, at the least, disciplinary actions by the Florida Board of Medicine for failing to obtain written consent before performing a pelvic exam*. The Florida mandates never define what exactly a "provider" is, and whether that individual could extend out to the limits of being a "provider" such as a registered nurse, a LVN (Limited Vocational Nurse), a Physician Assistant, a nurse's aide, a chiropractor, or perhaps even a massage therapist.

By the simple resurrection of Hippocrates, and the changing of the nondescript term "provider" to *physician*, perhaps the thinking of all those public forces may become more focused on the principles of Hippocrates.

And so that raises the question, why is there no mention of Hippocrates in these state efforts to define, control, and mandate every possible element of a "provider's" examination? Is any elected representative not aware of the Hippocratic Oath which specifically states the physician will be "avoiding any voluntary act of impropriety or corruption, including the seduction of women"—i.e., will not allow his or her physician human instincts to allow a deviation from the principles of ethical care? What is next on this increasingly lengthy and ill-advised agenda, signed consents for a breast exam with detailed definitions of what, actually, constitutes a breast examination, with a "gloved" hand, and with proscriptions about how much time may be expended examining each breast? Does an "escort" need to be present, what about a signed consent? What about a physician's effort required to physically move the left breast up or to the side, to facilitate the stethoscope examination of heart sounds...does that require a medical consent? Can the mouth be examined; can *anything* be examined without endless consent forms of the future?

I have heard physicians say that if patients (or State Legislatures) now start demanding a *witnessed signed consent agreement* for performing a Pap smear, they will strongly consider quitting the practice of medicine. On that matter, since the PAP smear to exclude cervical cancer is a routine element of a female's complete physical exam in my medical practice, I was often told *by the patient* that "an escort isn't needed, Doc, let's just get it over with, I trust you," and we'd proceed quickly and efficiently. In today's world, that kind of trust (both with the patient trusting the doctor to follow the Hippocratic mandates and the doctor equally trusting the patient not to make specious claims) has largely disappeared alongside the ethical lapses and the widely publicized lawsuits between doctors and patients. The female urology physician, assigned to check male urological organs, is another scenario that virtually never requires an "escort" to "assure propriety" during the examination—the rules are followed, the care is provided, and virtually all urological doctors regularly fulfill the expectations of Hippocrates.

All that aside, and even many years ago, precautions by physicians as well as their patients sometimes need to be taken. An interesting circumstance occurred a couple of years later, after the actress examination noted above, with a house call in a nearby wealthy community for a beautiful young female patient calling my office and asking for an examination for new and worrisome neurological complaints. She said she was unable to come to the office since she was feeling so sick, and I agreed to the house call as I have done for hundreds of other patients over the years. When her butler escorted me to the "massage room," where she was lying stark naked on the table and undergoing a therapeutic massage by a female Asian masseuse, I actually mentally thanked God that my young female medical assistant was standing (wide-eyed) right there at my side, available and ready to help in any way she could. As the masseuse rapidly lowered her head and scurried from the room, I carefully placed a towel over the patient and after gathering more history about her symptoms, I checked her physical and neurological condition. After I completed an appropriate neurological exam, I finally assured her that she was actually quite perfect and likely to live many more years without problems beyond those associated with her occasional anxiety and marital stress.

In this case, I felt the strong need for "plausible deniability" should any claim of impropriety take place...I trusted myself to do the right thing but I didn't fully trust the patient, and I therefore also ensured that I had an outstanding and trusted medical assistant at my side. During this entire process, there were no consent forms signed.

These two examples, extracted from the some of the years of my practice, give an indication of the potential circumstances where a doctor might be tempted to not follow the traditions established by the Hippocratic Oath if he or she adheres to less than the moral standards necessary for the ethical practice of medicine. Multiple other examples are present every day in a busy doctor's office—a prime example is the breast exam for tumors where there is nothing conveyed by the doctor during the exam beyond the concern about finding a small tumor which could end the patient's life if not identified. I made a decision in each case—the naked massage patient, for example, must have a female assistant with me during an exam while most other patients genuinely did not want or need more people crowding into the private examination room.

And so, with a name that has become as prominent as "Hippocrates," who was the man behind these standards, and how did his "oath" become emblazoned into our minds as we graduated from medical school? Of greatest practical importance, how did the Hippocratic standards and traditions become established as the bedrock of physician care?

Hippocrates was born about 460 BCE[44], on the Greek island of Kos (off the southern coast of Turkey). He was a Greek physician of the so-called Age of Pericles,[45] and he is considered one of the most outstanding figures in the history of medicine. The great philosopher, Plato, who lived around the same time, referred to him and his work in his writings, and the philosopher, Aristotle, also identified him as "The Great Physician" irrespective of the man's diminutive stature.[46] Hippocrates spent most of his life in Greece, and he is reported to have survived to the age of 83, 85, or 90 depending on what resource is reviewed.[47] Some say he lived to be more than 100[48] although there is little dependable information on the matter, and he finally expired in the ancient Greek region of Larissa, Thessaly (about 25 miles west of the Aegean Sea). He had two children, Thessalus and Draco, and in many ways, he lived a normal Greek life as a much-admired physician who traveled widely throughout Greece and much of Asia Minor, teaching students for a fee.

Although other men had practiced various elements of medicine helping afflicted patients prior to Hippocrates, the field of medical care had been enveloped in an aura of superstition, magic, and various supernatural elements that radiated voodoo concepts filled with religious rites. Hippocrates, however, turned a *science* concept into the reality of medical disease and is rightly thereby known as the Father of Modern Medicine. There is some controversy,[49] however, about whether Hippocrates himself actually wrote the oath that carries his name or whether it was a summary of ancient Greek writings that were associated with the work of this great physician. Also, it has been noted[50] that the original Greek version had to be translated into Latin first and then much later into English and other languages, and it is not certain what might have been lost in translation.

Although many of the teachings of Hippocrates about disease have been altered by scientific evolution and understanding, he was the first to describe important conditions that arose from disorders within the body. This directly contrasted from supernatural concepts that prevailed at that time. For example, he described the clubbing of fingers as indicating oxygen shortage (occasionally referred to as "Hippocratic fingers"),[51] linking a disease condition (chronic hypoxia or low oxygen level) with a physical finding. He regularly associated disease states with altered physiological conditions rather than voodoo-like alterations, and he developed many pulmonary (lung) procedures such as draining chest abscesses with a pipe (a treatment still being done today). One of the remarkable things about this is that he was able to perform much of these physiological interventions without the benefit of any detailed knowledge of anatomy, since dissections of humans in Greece were severely prohibited at that time.

Of greatest significance, however, was the legacy he created that defined the essential moral elements required of those who choose to practice medicine. Casting aside the human elements of sexuality, avarice and self-promotion, he portrayed the true physician to be an individual with the qualities of honesty and compassion, while maintaining honorable principles while caring for a patient. These beliefs then became embodied in the most famous medical treatise ever developed in the history of the world and enshrined for thousands of years thereafter: the Hippocratic Oath. Written as a guidance that mandated doctors must uphold the covenants essential to practicing the art of medicine, always working on the behalf of patients, the oath outlines an ethical doctor's behavior. Following is the original Hippocratic Oath:

I swear by Apollo the physician, and Asclepius, and Hygieia and Panacea and all the gods and goddesses as my witnesses, that, according to my ability and judgement, I will keep this Oath and this contract:

To hold him who taught me this art equally dear to me as my parents, to be a partner in life with him, and to fulfill his needs when required; to look upon his offspring as equals to my own siblings, and to teach them this art, if they shall wish to learn it, without fee or contract; and that by the set rules, lectures, and every other mode of instruction, I will impart a knowledge of the art to my own sons, and those of my teachers, and to students bound by this contract and having sworn this Oath to the law of medicine, but to no others.

I will use those dietary regimens which will benefit my patients according to my greatest ability and judgement, and I will do no harm or injustice to them.

I will not give a lethal drug to anyone if I am asked, nor will I advise such a plan; and similarly I will not give a woman a pessary to cause an abortion.

In purity and according to divine law will I carry out my life and my art.

I will not use the knife, even upon those suffering from stones, but I will leave this to those who are trained in this craft.

Into whatever homes I go, I will enter them for the benefit of the sick, avoiding any voluntary act of impropriety or corruption, including the seduction of women or men, whether they are free men or slaves.

Whatever I see or hear in the lives of my patients, whether in connection with my professional practice or not, which ought not to be spoken of outside, I will keep secret, as considering all such things to be private.

So long as I maintain this Oath faithfully and without corruption, may it be granted to me to partake of life fully and the practice of my art, gaining the respect of all men for all time. However, should I transgress this Oath and violate it, may the opposite be my fate.

History of Medicine Division
National Library of Medicine
National Institutes of Health

Alterations in this oath have been proposed by numerous entities, and as many as 7 different versions have been widely distributed. These versions include one that changes the original oath to a shorter oath that was endorsed by a Geneva Convention. Another one, a "Modern Hippocratic Oath" was drawn up by Dr. Louis

Lasagna in 1964 and has found widespread use for graduating medical school classes. Yet another one, a Russian version, was approved by the "Supreme Soviet USSR" (in 1971), and there was the "Oath of the Healer" created by Louis Weinstein, and *another* oath became generated that curiously, "Bears the Name of Hippocrates."[52] Finally, a tiny postscript-like "Code of Ethics" commentary by the American Medical Association was offered to be used after 1980.[53] Many of the changes have been stimulated by those who simply want to shorten it, to change its ancient dialogue, to simplify it, or simply to bring about a change by those who take exception to some of the original specific recommendations.

Louis Lasagna's "Modern Version," in 2001, gives perhaps one of the best modifications of the original:

I swear to fulfill, to the best of my ability and judgment, this covenant: I will respect the hard-won scientific gains of those physicians in whose steps I walk, and gladly share such knowledge as is mine with those who are to follow.

I will apply, for the benefit of the sick, all measures [that] are required, avoiding those twin traps of overtreatment and therapeutic nihilism.

I will remember that there is art to medicine as well as science, and that warmth, sympathy, and understanding may outweigh the surgeon's knife or the chemist's drug.

I will not be ashamed to say "I know not," nor will I fail to call in my colleagues when the skills of another are needed for a patient's recovery.

I will respect the privacy of my patients, for their problems are not disclosed to me that the world may know. Most especially must I tread with care in matters of life and death. If it is given me to save a life, all thanks. But it may also be within my power to take a life; this awesome responsibility must be faced with great humbleness and awareness of my own frailty. Above all, I must not play at God.

I will remember that I do not treat a fever chart, a cancerous growth, but a sick human being, whose illness may affect the person's family and economic stability. My responsibility includes these related problems, if I am to care adequately for the sick.

I will prevent disease whenever I can, for prevention is preferable to cure.

I will remember that I remain a member of society, with special obligations to all my fellow human beings, those sound of mind and body as well as the infirm.

If I do not violate this oath, may I enjoy life and art, respected while I live and remembered with affection thereafter. May I always act so as to preserve the finest traditions of my calling and may I long experience the joy of healing those who seek my help.[54]

Dr. Sherman Mellinkoff, the former Dean of the UCLA School of Medicine, provided an oath for the school's graduating medical students, taken by hundreds of students, including myself. Following is the oath, which I spoke in 1975 and was recited again this year by the graduating class of UCLA's David Geffen School of Medicine:

I swear by all that I hold most sacred that I will keep this enduring Oath:

To the best of my ability and judgment I will practice the Art only for the benefit of my patients.

Whatever houses I may visit, I will enter only to help the sick or to prevent illness, never to inflict harm, injustice or suffering.

I will lead my life and practice the Art conscientiously and with honor.

Whatever I may see or hear in the practice of the Art, or even outside of it that should not be spread abroad, I will keep in solemn confidence.

I will be just and generous to those who taught me the Art, to my colleagues in the Art, and to those who desire to learn it.

May happiness and the physician's good repute be granted me while I keep this sacred Oath inviolate.[55]

And as the Oath has undergone evolutions, the multiple versions have regularly created a mandate for the following primary principles:

1. I will practice my art of medicine solely to help my patients.

2. I will enter the private arena of those patients to provide that help and to never create any harmful consequences.
3. I will be conscientious and honorable as I practice the art of medicine.
4. I will never divulge secrets of patients.
5. I will assist and teach my colleagues to the best of my ability.
6. I will adhere to this Hippocratic Code, and I will consider it sacred.

These concepts surround the longstanding primary guiding principle for doctors: *primum non nocere*, (First, Do No Harm). The Latin wording of this powerful statement is not in the Hippocratic Oath, *per se*, since the oath is in Greek, although it is suspected that similar wording we see today in translated versions evolved from another of Hippocratic's works called *Of the Epidemics*.[56] However, as noted, many medical schools have created their own oaths that reflect various philosophical sentiments of their authors. An example of this is found at the University of California, San Francisco, where students vow not to discriminate against patients based on gender, race, religion, or sexual orientation. Further extensions of perceived bias continue to move into various oaths in an effort to ensure all discrimination against any human being for any reason will be addressed. Missing from the more "modern" versions of this oath are the considerations of giving a lethal drug or taking actions which would cause abortions, both of which actions may be legally initiated today by doctors, depending on state law. The providing of pain or anxiety-relieving drugs to suffering patients with terminal diseases in high dosages, potentially causing an earlier death, is not discussed. Also missing may be anything specifically relating to the seduction of "men or women" in the course of doctor activities; requiring doctors to be "conscientious and honorable" is perhaps close enough to the same thing.

Although the vast majority of American physicians strongly believe in these basic principles, there has been a diminishment in the *application* of the Hippocratic Oath, especially in the past 50 years. This decline has not followed any intentional pathway of diabolical intent, but rather has been the unfortunate consequence of altering standards in the delivery of healthcare. The result of this is, unfortunately, closely related to the disappearance of available primary care physicians for patients who have a need for decent care; it is notable that Hippocrates, by most standards, lived his professional life like a primary care physician, while setting standards for all doctors.

The beginning of this decline might be seen by the shrinking numbers of graduating physicians requested to speak this oath at the time of their commencement ceremonies at medical school, although presumably, most of the students are intrinsically aware of the oath and are willing to follow its moral mandates. The dropping percentage of these graduating students taking the oath is now to a degree that should alarm anybody trying to obtain decent primary care. Currently, approximately only 11% of medical students currently speak the *classic* Hippocratic Oath, although a survey (in 2009) revealed with some encouragement that 33% still recite Lasagna's Oath (the "Modern Version")[57] at their graduation. Looking at all of the doctors in the United States, another study[58] found that a grand total of 56% of physicians spoke *some kind of* Hippocratic Oath at their graduation ceremony. Furthermore, as evidence of decline from the original mandates in the oath, euthanasia is prohibited in only 14% of the various spoken oaths, while only 8% prohibit abortion, and only 3% of the oaths specifically prohibit sexual contact with patients.[59] It has also been observed[60] that, while the original Hippocratic Oath calls for "the opposite" of pleasure and fame for anybody who violates the oath, less than half of today's oaths define this punishment or accountability for digressing from its moral mandates.

There should be a national concern asking the question why barely half of the doctors in the United States give verbal recognition of the principles critical to the essence of the Hippocratic Oath. Can the half of our doctor population who *do not* speak or give any recognition to this oath still be counted on by the patients in our country to provide care that conforms to the highest ethical standards? As the thousands of years have passed since the Hippocratic Oath first evolved (and became recognized as an inviolate oath by emerging physicians), the evolution and modernization of our society has promoted an atmosphere of disregard for the oath, irrespective of the moral absolutes within. The consequences of this irrelevance have been profound to the practice of medicine and more recently, to the numbers of available physicians who may continue practicing this previously honored profession. And, it is worth noting that, nowhere, in all of the writings from Hippocrates is there any mention of a "provider" rather than a doctor.

The largest purported "representative" organization for medical doctors, the American Medical Association (AMA), might be expected to define, and give order to, this increasingly disordered ethical evolution. And yet, a declining number of physicians actually belong to this organization which is so often quoted in news reports as "representing the physicians of America." The drop in membership has been a profound disgrace to the once proud organization. In the 1950s, 75% of doctors were AMA members and there was a generally united approach to national matters of medical importance, including the Hippocratic Oath. However, over the years, as political rhetoric in our country became increasingly toxic, the AMA has angered members more and more until the membership in this organization plummeted down now to less than 25%.[61] And once a doctor leaves the AMA, there is little chance the organization may bring him back. The additional reasons for this decline are many and complex, but many observers believe the progressively liberal nature of the organization, including their more recent support for ObamaCare while endorsing numerous other liberal political positions desired by the federal government, has alienated much of its membership.

In the political spectrum of doctors in America, conflicting data has demonstrated a climbing number of Democrat physicians currently caring for patients compared with previous years. A 2016 Gallup poll[62] found that 35% of doctors considered themselves Democrats while 27% were Republicans and 36% identified as independents; by 2018, nearly two-thirds of physician campaign contributions went to Democrats while one-third went to Republicans[63] which may help explain the liberal nature of the organization's leadership. Factors affecting this include increasing numbers of females graduating from medical school (currently about 50%), since females are reportedly more likely to be Democrats,[64] and increasing numbers of physicians working for managed care entities rather than private practices, a process that reduces the number of physician business owners (who are more frequently considered to be Republican oriented).

However, many physicians have reported[65] over the past 20 years that if the AMA could simply endorse the principles of decent healthcare, so well defined in the Hippocratic Oath, and not deviate back and forth with other positions across the political spectrum, the organization might be seen as providing a better representation of the American doctor. If that is a future possibility, it is hoped the membership numbers may climb again and true representation of the American physician might again emerge. Considering the huge variation of physicians' political positions, however, it would be very unlikely a single organization could adequately represent the doctors of America before the public and Congress, unless politics were removed from the national medical sentiments, an unlikely proposition.

There are many other types of gatherings of physicians, including state medical organizations, Hispanic medical organizations, the Doctors without Borders organization, an Indian Academy of Pediatrics Doctors, and many other specialty and subspecialty organizations. This potpourri of medical organizations are often non-persuasive in the political arena because of their limited clout. This ineffectiveness in generating political policy has added to the reasons why it has become nearly impossible to generate laws and public policies that solidify moral standards and create a renewed possibility of increased numbers of new primary care physicians for the American population.

Perhaps a new physician organization, something called "Hippocrates Medical Association" would draw a significant number of primary care physicians who place the quality and standards of care above all else. One organization that seems to be focused on proper care for patients, Physicians for Patient Protection, reportedly[66] has more than 12,000 physician members and is showing promise for returning proper focus to the Hippocratic Oath model of decent patient care.

As the numbers of available physicians providing primary care to the patients of our communities have declined, and if what is left of "organized medicine" does not seem to notice, the revered tradition of bedside manner suffers profoundly. A bedside manner *takes time and it takes effort.* The doctor at the bedside in a patient's home, the doctor sitting next to a patient in his or her hospital room, the doctor in his office have all largely disappeared with ever-shrinking available time and patient volume overload, creating an increasing evolution of a robotic-like state of doctor personae. A doctor who rushes into a hospitalized patient's room and asks hurried questions followed by a cursory exam has failed the basic tenants of decent bedside manner and care established in traditions spanning thousands of years.

People may have loved their doctors in the days gone by, but it is difficult to love a doctor's computer which continuously sits in front of the doctor and seems to constantly compete for attention. The proliferation of computers has stimulated this change, as computers have expanded the challenging evolutions in our social media, even while making information more readily available. Computers in our society have changed what people say to each other, how often they may react negatively to whatever seems to increasingly offend, and for the doctor, it has resulted in a computer screen that often interferes with the crucial pathway between the doctor's eyes and the patient's face. "He spends more time looking at his computer screen than listening to me!" has been an ever-increasing patient complaint, with the attendant loss of the precious human interaction that would otherwise promote trust in the doctor's capabilities and humanity. Interestingly, with the Covid mandates, this same concept has been expressed in businesses that have expanded Zoom interactions with similar loss of the vital human element so vital to social and business interactions.

When a doctor hears a female patient say something like, "Doctor, at home, I'm beginning to feel the pain of our marriage," and he types on his computer patient record, or records into his transcribing machine, "Patient unhappy with husband," the entire doctor-patient-empathy component has disappeared. And without empathy, many patients may ask, can there *really* be understanding? Empathy can drain a doctor when he or she is called upon to understand stressful emotional circumstances, over and over throughout the day, and yet the energies that goes into that drain are necessary components for the understanding of a patient's needs. Finally, the patient may ask himself or herself as she eventually leaves the doctor's office, "Did he even *begin* to understand my home situation? Is it possible that he is going to help me?" And, finally, "Should I consider changing doctors?"

Why do doctors look at computer screens while the patient is talking? The computers are obviously a more efficient way to gather information in a time-challenged office, to look at lab, to look at x-ray reports, to see historical facts and to review consulting doctors' input, the doctor hoping to find trends and other indicators that might aid a diagnosis. Doctors will tell you it helps with their efficiency. But, what is the *next* step if the patient is becoming merely a voice in the computerized background? Like a Zoom session, maybe? Or, could this activity eventually expand to just a recording from the patient to be automatically entered into the computer? As our technological capabilities with artificial intelligence expand, can the computer develop a treatment plan, finally printing outpatient instructions?

While these activities may be an "efficient" way to conduct a medical practice and to save time when the schedule is packed, is it a good thing when the treasured tradition of the doctor's bedside manner is lost? Can it be considered that, when the patient has moved into an examining room, *then* that may be a good time for the doctor to quickly dictate a note that summarizes the essence of the patient's concerns? If the time-crunch did not create such a driving force for efficiency at the expense of human relationships, wouldn't a doctor putting the computer aside for a few minutes to really *listen* to the patient be a good idea? And, when the doctor rushes into the exam room and quickly checks the patient's heart, often through time-efficient multiple layers of clothing, is that an adequate examination? A subtle yet diagnostic heart murmur can adequately be heard through interfering layers of shirt and undershirt? Finally, when the examination does take place, are the patient's important signs of clammy hands, a slight tremor, the anxious look in the eyes, the averted gaze, or the faint bead of sweat on the brow, going to be missed and discarded in concert with the efficiency of the quick exam? Running behind schedule, with patients streaming into the waiting room, if the doctor would just spend a few minutes more to help sustain such important elements of the doctor-patient contact, while improving communications and care, all of it would make Hippocrates proud.

And the pathway to a happier and healthier patient may then become re-established as the traditions from Hippocrates become, once again, the centerpiece of American medicine.

Chapter 4

The Drugs

To talk about drugs is to talk about life.

The spectrum of human experience with all that creates our moods, our sufferings, our pleasures, and even our survivability has existed since the beginning of humanity. From the earliest days of the human race to the creation of the behemoth pharmaceutical industry of today, drugs have affected this spectrum positively and negatively. In more modern times, as the underlying mechanism of disease became better understood, drugs regularly save lives (e.g. antibiotics) while improving lives (Viagra, antidepressants, caffeine, and analgesics) and reducing risks of death (statin cholesterol reducers, anti-hypertensives, diabetes medications and modern cardiac medications). It is easy to presume that the needs for the vast array of drugs in use today is mostly a modern phenomenon, and yet the same needs for these medications existed not only back in the beginning of recorded time, but ever more extensively during the evolution of civilization, including Hippocrates' Greek society. The need has continued throughout the earliest days of the developing Asian civilization, through the development of civilizations in Europe and America, and continuing all the way to life today. This need has cultivated, in parallel, a pharmacologic industry that has expanded exponentially into a world of megapharmacies linked with insurance systems, financial controlling systems, and a human population that craves not just survival and relief of pain and suffering but also pleasure mixed with a powerful need for satisfaction in all the arenas of life.

It is clear, therefore, that the craving of our population for these drug solutions is not just a modern phenomenon. As Hippocrates travelled throughout his world in Greece that existed circa 400 BC, he certainly recognized these same human needs from the patients as they individually and collectively pleaded with him for a better (and longer) life, each patient looking to this remarkable physician to provide answers. And there were answers, although Hippocrates was one of the earliest medical doctors to clearly separate superstitions and gods from human illness which he identified to be caused by natural forces.[67] Probably one of the greatest contributions of Hippocrates to the evolving understanding of medication was, therefore, to separate human need from religion, and to identify that humans required medication not because of a punishment inflicted by the gods but because of environmental factors (bacteria and viruses unknown at that time), as well as to bring some chance of a longer survival after a lifetime of harm from the forces of nature, marginal diets and poor living habits. It is remarkable, considering the general beliefs of his day, that nowhere in his extensive writings (the *Hippocratic Corpus*),[68] is there any mention of mystical illnesses. Furthermore, he did not focus on medications as solutions to human illness and he exhibited a reluctance to administer drugs that might be wrongly chosen...often defaulting to recommendations that included fasting saying, "to eat when you are sick, is to feed your sickness."[69] The Hippocratic drug program was, therefore, highly limited and he often prescribed, with fasting, a simple mixture of honey and vinegar, using more potent drugs only on rare specific occasions.

When drugs were considered to be of potential help in those Greek times, what medication was actually available? Herbal "medications" had been used for the entire spectrum of human need, and a vast array of sources was available[70] including such herbs as Oregano, Mountain Tea (Tsai Tou Vounou), Lemon Balm, Bay Leaf, Mastic Tree, St. John's Wort, and Sage. However, the most powerful medications of those days were Opium and Hemp (or "charred hemp, the source of cannabis or marijuana). Opium's effects were known long before Hippocrates, dating back to the earliest days of civilization, including even the Assyrians (in 2500 BC, during the time of Mesopotamia) who referred to the poppy as the "Happy Plant." Egyptian tombs contained jugs of opium residue, and there are ancient descriptions[71] of the pain-relieving (and even life-ending) effects of the drug.

Hemp has a longer history than even opium, remarkably evolving (without human presence) 28 million years ago on the eastern Tibetan Plateau,[72] according to a recent pollen study. Looking at geological formations on our planet, the oldest large-scale stretch of opium-compatible ancient surface lies in the Negev Desert, "just" 1.8 million years old.[73] Human civilization (that is, *Homo sapiens*, evolving from *Homo erectus* and migrating out of

Africa about 300,000 years ago)[74] has been documented to have existed in central Europe for just the past 5,000 years. Chinese mourners burned cannabis for its intoxicating fumes on a remote mountain plateau in Central Asia some 2500 years ago,[75] one of the earliest documentations of the drug used for pharmacologic use (in this case, the relief of grief during a mourning ceremony). The Romans knew about this drug as evidenced by the tomb of a 14-yr-old girl who apparently died while giving birth (found in the 1990s near Jerusalem)...a substance in the child's skeletal abdominal area was analyzed and found to be tetrahydrocannabinol, a component of cannabis, presumably used to relieve the girl of pain and, perhaps, even to relieve her of life itself. Finally, as we move ahead throughout the centuries of drug use, it is estimated[76] that 150 million people regularly smoke cannabis today for its touted medical and psychological effects.

And so, following this evolution of drugs from Mesopotamia through Roman Times, through Chinese evolutions and throughout the time of the Greek civilization and Hippocrates, what has happened in our society with drugs as we look at the world in which we live today?

This subject of drugs in the United States has generated more analysis, more hostility, more political divisiveness, more reverence, more regulation, and even more appreciation than virtually any other element in our society. Of course, the term "drugs" evokes images of drug-addicted people dying of variable consequences of their chemical cravings and dependence, and that effect is certainly demonstrated on a regular basis. In the spectrum that includes legalized drugs as well as "street" drugs, ranging from alcohol to marijuana, from morphine to heroin, from Viagra to Ecstasy, birth control pills as well as medications to induce abortion, LSD, and beyond, millions of hours of legal debates have been generated, periods of national prohibition have been instituted, and endless discussions about the good and bad of these substances have raged across our country. While this debate continues to flourish, a wide spectrum of drugs jam the shelves of our drugstores, displaying a vast quantity of over-the-counter chemical and vitamin substances of variable, and often questionable, benefit for a suffering patient.

That leads to the question asking which individual drugs are "good" and which drugs are "bad?" *It depends on who is doing the looking*, the patient, the doctor, the pharmacist, the insurance company, or even the law enforcement agencies of our country.

This arena of chemicals available to the public is vast, with currently over 20,000 prescription drug products[77] available for those who are determined to have a need. As a doctor prescribing for my patients, I look at drugs in terms of risk and benefit, and always with cost considerations. As a patient, however, I can look at the same drug and place benefit as more important than risk or cost. Same drug, completely different perspective. Like beauty is in the eyes of the beholder, the considerations about drugs' effects being beautiful or ugly depend on the perspective of the individual doing the looking. Also, it follows that whether a drug is "good" or "bad" in the eyes of doctors is different from the vision of pharmacists, from the view of the police and our legal system, that of pharmaceutical CEO's, of drug rehab centers, of parents (or their children), of attorneys, of Democrats or Republicans, of the wealthy and the impoverished, of medical insurance companies and their adjusters, overseers of Medicare and/or Medicaid, and the drug monitoring directors within the Veterans Administration.

The vast arena of drug observers not only have opinions about prescription drugs, there has also been substantial effort to control the distribution of many drugs, as well as the cost of the drugs, the availability, the utilization, and even the patterns of drug consumption. It often starts with a patient having symptoms who sees his or her doctor and it is determined that a medication is needed. The doctor is licensed and *most of the time*, the medication is going to be appropriate for the patient's condition although this (on rare occasions) may not always be the case.

One of the more flagrant examples of a doctor's prescription being a bad plan in our community was demonstrated by a physician in our community who was widely known by Emergency Room doctors as "the Candy Man" (before he was sent to prison for an extended time). For the sake of money, he abandoned all the ethics that may have come to him in earlier days from the moralities of Hippocrates as well as the rules of medical societies, licensing mandates and legal regulations. He provided thousands of prescriptions for pharmacologic substances to make his habituated patients happy while satisfying their addictive cravings. The Candy Man considered these drugs to be good (especially since the drug consumer would pay him handsomely for them), the patients craving the drugs considered them to be wonderful, the ER doctors looked at the drugs and the doctor with disgust (as they treated numerous overdose consequences), and the legal system (after an inexplicably long delay) determined that his whole prescribing pattern was illegal and bad, very bad, and then put the doctor away in prison. The fact that, at the same time, this doctor also lost his license suggests that the Medical Board of California considered this drug distribution pattern to be unethical and in violation of the standards for licensure.

So, when a doctor follows a Hippocratic pathway and prescribes a drug for a patient, it would seem that a relatively straightforward trail would lead to the purchase and the ingestion of the drug. Until a few years ago, this pathway was not complex. The patient would take the prescription to the pharmacist and would then purchase a bottle or vial of medication leading to, hopefully, a favorable resolution of symptoms and improvement of the condition. But as the number of available medications expanded by the tens of thousands, the landscape became filled with ever-increasing masses of entrepreneurs inserted into this otherwise direct pathway. Money, greed, regulatory power, and competition all played a role in this evolving caldron of disruption that has increasingly brought so much harm to the good process of a pharmacist filling a prescription for a suffering patient. These forces include the skyrocketing cost of new drugs, the worldwide production of generic substitutes, the expanding insurance industry that controls so much of the pricing that will be passed on to the patient, and the ever-variable premiums paid for this control. On top of all that, there is the Federal Drug Administration, with their thousands of regulations that try to control drugs, the wholesalers who have become titans at altering the costs of drugs, the pharmaceutical companies who have replaced quality pharmacist counsel and advice for distribution volume, and finally the myriad of companies who have inserted themselves into this entire debacle of drug administration.

It is important to note that the setting of cost is not controlled by the government or any regulatory agency. The company *making* the drug, the pharmaceutical company, together with all the additional layers of cost-generating factors, determine the initial cost for a pharmacy to purchase the drug for distribution, this purchase reflecting the following variables:

- How competitive the drug is likely to be
- The molecular mechanism of drug effects and mechanism of action
- The drug's uniqueness compared to other drugs already on the market
- The effectiveness of the drug against often complex diseases
- The cost of trials utilizing an adequate number of patients (together with a control group), both under "blinded" circumstances, to allow final FDA approval after confirming statistical significance of benefit

- The side-effects of the drug on patients in the trial and the legal risks from these side-effects
- The costs of drug manufacturing

When a patient looks at a new prescription, he or she generally thinks only three things: will the drug help the problem, will there be any side-effects that could cause harm, and how much will the drug cost? The first two questions depend largely on the competence and training of the medical doctor as well as the pharmaceutical testing process that establishes risk and benefit. How much will the drug cost is the question that will take the patient onto a road that is filled with some of the most avaricious manipulators of drug acquisition and pricing that would have shocked and horrified Hippocrates.

A patient might wonder as he or she ponders the cost of a drug, would it be worth the effort to look to the insurance company for guidance about payment for the drug? This would seem logical, since insurance companies are often called upon to cover much of the payments for drugs, and such an inquiry would be especially important with the more expensive ones. However, since the insurance company's policy makers do in fact control payment for patients' drugs, (and determining which brand-name versus generic drugs are "allowed"), this is a process that often amounts to controlling the drug distribution from American drug manufacturers as well as controlling the massive distribution of generic drugs from countries like China and India, like generic drugs from Lupin Drugs made in Dubai, India? Or from *Farmacias Similares* in Mexico? They are *really* FDA approved? Can I trust the FDA? Can I trust these drugs?

With my father's digitalis, for example, the insurance company clearly stated they would cover some of the cost of a generic drug while they would not cover the cost of the exact same chemical that was a brand-name drug. And the generic drug they would cover may be the same chemical but manufactured where, a patient might wonder? In the middle of all this debate, generic drug manufacturers revealed that the high price of brand-name drugs made it nearly impossible for them to purchase enough drugs for generic developments and testing, delaying the generic drug competition for the pharmaceutical company, even as the drug's patent ran out. A sizable portion of generic drugs do come from India (dominating the generic drugs market, exporting nearly $20 billion worth of drugs per year...20% of the global market) and China which has 230 of the nearly 2,000 manufacturing sites in the world.[78] Of the "essential" drugs (like anesthetics, antibacterial, antidepressant, antiviral, cardiovascular and gastrointestinal agents) 21% are still made in the United States while 15% are from China; clearly, although both China and India export sizable amounts of generic drugs to the United States, neither is dominant over the supply from the remainder of the world.

Finally, as the company's directors continued to point at the Research and Development costs as the main driver of cost, it was revealed that the drug company Teva's $689 million in development costs since 1989 was only about 2% of the company's U.S. profits from 2002 to 2019; Teva is the world's largest generic drug manufacturer, producing more than 120 billion tablets with one in nine generic prescriptions in the US containing the company's products. Finally, the investigation found that "the single-greatest step to curb prices would be to allow Medicare to negotiate prices." The companies under investigation indicated that the noncompetitive U.S. market — specifically with Medicare — was the means to ensure high profits.

This decision-making capability introduces the concept of profit through the process of mandating a very cheap generic drug creating billions of dollars of profit—while purportedly looking to protect the patient from excessive expenditures. The insurance companies are, first and foremost, looking to protect their own company's profit as they endeavor to hold the line on competitive insurance premiums for their customers (the patients). From a financial standpoint, all of this seems good and that the patient would benefit...and so it is worth looking at the payments for medication, where they go, who gathers up all the money the patient pays (either directly as the drug is purchased, or indirectly through insurance premiums).

But first, unfortunately, it is important to recognize that it is not just the insurance company that sets the patient's cost for drugs and it is not a simple matter of dictating costs for brand-name versus generic. In reality, there is a significant number of other companies that have inserted themselves in-between the doctor, the prescription, the pharmacy, and the patient. This includes, remarkably, the ever-expanding Medicare and Medicaid government bureaucrats, it includes the giant wholesalers AmerisourceBergen, Cardinal, and McKesson, it includes the pharmacists' migraine-inducing nightmare that nobody ever heard of called "Pharmacy Benefit Management" (PBM), it includes an egregious added fee attachment called the Direct and Indirect Remuneration (DIR) Fee, and it includes the computer-dependent drug-purchasing systems like PBM-controlled GoodRx with their printable coupons. This DIR fee is, if you can stretch your imagination, a cover-all term that allows "the monies that a Medicare Part D plan may collect to offset member costs."[79] All of these entities have been able to insert themselves into the seemingly simple relationship of doctor-prescription-pharmacy-patient.

Our country is then filled with a gigantic morass of differing drug perspectives and control patterns. And each of these categories of observers and controllers have subsets, and more subsets of the subsets, all together creating a vast universe of drug payment activity that can overwhelm the observer's previous understanding about the profit-motives of drug distribution as well as the previous consideration of the cost of a drug to help a patient. This chaos of the human element is so much more complex than the scientific studies that carefully apply controlled trials looking at statistical data to determine the good and the bad of any drug substance, studies that hopefully remove all bias that may exist in the observer. Because of these trials and the observations of entities as divergent as the government's Medicare ICD-10 billing creators, the syphoning of money by PBM and computer-stimulated coupon-printing forces of GoodRx, as well as the DIR fee, contrasts sharply with physicians who have to make drug decisions as their patients who are sitting or lying before them with desperate needs. And, in a reflection of the doctor-patient relationship, the final determination of a drug being good or bad or even available often diminishes the emotional element of trust for the doctor that might otherwise be felt by the patient. And this kind of trust is not just for receiving a drug, it is the trust in the physician *prescribing the drug* that is so inherent in the doctor-patient bond that has existed since Hippocrates.

Looking back at Hippocrates again for a better perspective, and contrasting with the tens of thousands of prescription drugs that are available today, which medicines beyond herbs, charred hemp and opium were available to the physicians at that time? Struggling with the absence of knowledge about internal organs and their interrelationships, as well as the absence of knowledge about bacteria and viruses, medications that could affect these organs or the invading bacterial pathogens had not yet been discovered. Drugs were given to make the patient feel better...inherent with this concept was the hope that the patient might not die from their diseases *because drugs were given*. Also, there was a concern that a potential death from drugs during the time of Hippocrates easily included death *induced by the drug itself*. And since the fundamental healing ability of the human body was felt by Hippocrates to be the result of the "healing powers of nature," his therapeutic approach was based on the ability of the patient to rebalance the essential and fundamental "four humours" consisting of black bile, blood, phlegm, and yellow bile.

These four elements were not just contrived or invented, they were the direct result of observing a tube of fresh blood that had been watched after an hour or so. Layers appeared, a dark clot forming at the bottom (black bile), above the clot was a layer of red cells (blood), above that was a pale layer of white blood cells (the phlegm), and on the top was the clear yellow serum (yellow bile). Since everybody's blood demonstrated those four layers, it seemed likely that they controlled the patient's disease-fighting processes, and that "the healing power of nature" would come from the best medication available. The result of this philosophy was a reluctance to administer *any* drug substances beyond honey and vinegar with the hope that the patient's body itself could re-balance the four humours and heal. Wound treatment in the time of Hippocrates then consisted of using "clean" water or wine on wounds, and occasional soothing balms.[80] As I have noted, only on rare occasions did Hippocrates use more potent drugs.[81] With that safe policy, the actual *killing* of a patient from taking a drug would be a rare event and the doctors of the time would feel safe.

When my father was struggling to breathe on that stormy day of his desperate call, he did not know that what he was really seeking was just two drugs: digitalis and a diuretic. Furthermore, his disease condition, that of a failing heart, was not unique to modern times in our country, it was a failure of cardiac strength (from many possible causes) that pleaded for just these two medicines. He did not know that concept, however, and all he knew for sure was that he was going to die soon if his condition provoking his shortness of breath continued to worsen. If he had lived in the time of Hippocrates, it would have been resoundingly evident that providing Opium or charred Hemp would not have done much beyond slowing his breathing and giving him a relatively peaceful death. And when I finally was able to get him into the hospital, digitalis and diuretics were quickly administered *intravenously* with a life-saving benefit that was expected by his cardiac physician, and was remarkable to everyone else. However, without the availability of these prescription drugs, he had no way of obtaining critically needed treatment, even if he knew of their names, underscoring the critical link between his prescribing physician (who was unavailable that weekend) and a very sick patient needing a critical drug.

It is notable that the recognition of digitalis evolved well before modern times. When did research first discover this life-saving drug from the tall and stately Foxglove plant known as Digitalis lanata? This plant's dried leaf is the source of the medicine, and the plant's name has morphed into a more descriptive title of *Digitalis Purpurea*. The leaves, the flowers and the seeds of this plant are all poisonous to humans if taken in sufficient quantity although recorded Foxglove poisonings are very rare. Although the drug was unknown during the time of Hippocrates, Digitalis has been known since the early days of the American Revolution, discovered in 1775,[82] and it then subsequently became recognized as a drug that could help failing hearts. The English physician William Withering is credited with the first published description of the use of Digitalis derivatives in his 1785 book *An Account of The Foxglove and Some of Its Medical Uses With Practical Remarks on Dropsy and Other Diseases*.[83] Now available as Digoxin, carrying the brand name Lanoxin, the drug stimulates the cardiac muscle to contract more vigorously to push excess fluid (that has backed into the lungs causing the shortness-of-breath) down into the kidneys where it may be excreted, often aided by a diuretic to push the fluid into the bladder and then out of the body. This removal of excess fluid then helps the heart and relieves the symptoms of congestive heart failure.

Of greater significance is the evolution and spectrum of cost to patients for this plant's pharmacologic property. As an older drug, having been discovered hundreds of years ago, and as a drug readily created by a plant, Digoxin would seem to be cheap, almost free, easily prescribed, and readily available. Grow the plant, extract the drug, easy. Remarkably, the seed company Burpee has even extensive Foxglove cultivating instructions on its website and it even offers free shipping to anybody who wants to grow the plants in a garden. To the company's credit, it does note the poisonous nature of the Foxglove plant, and there are no recommendations for gardeners to try it for its medicinal effects.

Going back to the beginning of congestive heart failure symptoms, it is worth looking into what a patient could experience if his or her doctor provided a prescription for Lanoxin. The Rx would read something like, "Lanoxin, 0.125 mg. sig. 1 q AM PO, qs 30 days, refill x2." Translated, this would be instructions to the pharmacist to fill a small plastic container in the drugstore with 30 Brand Name Digoxin pills having a strength of 0.125 milligrams with instructions to take one by mouth each morning, and to then provide two refills for a total of three months of medication.

With the prescription in hand after leaving the doctor's office, the patient would seek a pharmacy to fill the prescription. He or she would not necessarily think about the cost since the shortness-of-breath was frightening and a sense of impending mortality kept arising in the patient's mind...this was clearly an essential drug and cost compared to survival would not be a deciding factor. However, with a sense of due diligence, there was a need to check local prices at the nearby pharmacies.

Since life was certainly at risk, the thought of checking the computer and buying the original patented drug (Lanoxin) rather than a cheaper generic drug (digoxin) seemed reasonable. But, what would the price be? Looking for Lanoxin sources on the internet, the patient found the patent-holding company was GlaxoSmithKline, the drug was manufactured by Advanz Pharma Corp, a multi-national pharmaceutical company headquartered in London, recently changing its name from Concordia Healthcare Corporation. None of that seemed to matter, but the cost of a one month supply of the drug ranged from $440* at Costco to $455 at Vons and Albertsons, and $463 at CVS. These prices were available if a coupon from an internet company GoodRx, was to be used, and the website conveniently made such price comparisons available. As the patient was increasingly short-of-breath, he or she would then find that if an injectable drug would be given for a faster result, the cost was $1,210 for a little less than 10 *liquid* doses...only enough for about 1/3 month. But the doctor had definitely provided a prescription that instructed the Lanoxin will be *pills* to be taken by mouth, not injectable, leading to further research which showed the medicine

* All prices are at the time of this manuscript development, drug prices from different pharmacies change with time.

was available as a pill for a three month supply: the cost for 100 pills would be $1513.00. The advantage of a three month supply, however, would be that the symptoms might clear for a longer time and the patient wouldn't have to run back for refills. However, the prescription specifically said one month, not three months, and two refills were ordered.

It was noted that my father, who was finally quickly hospitalized at our local hospital, actually received intravenous digoxin initially, costing him at least $120 per dose.

The next thought for the patient seeking Lanoxin was an encouraging one: how much would the drug cost *if it was covered by insurance* since the patient was already paying thousands of dollars per year for the coverage by a decent insurance policy? And also, since the patient was in the Medicare system, shouldn't this government medical program for the elderly population cover drugs, especially essential long-established cardiac drugs like Lanoxin? A quick call to the insurance company confirmed, after waiting nearly an hour on-hold and listening to a long string of near-useless recordings, that the brand name would definitely *not* be covered and the patient must purchase the generic drug only to have insurance coverage. They repeated it twice, under no circumstance would the brand name be covered. So, encouraged by that news that at least *something* would be covered, all that was needed now was to inform the pharmacy that insurance and Medicare was available and the generic form would be purchased. With that, what would the cost now be, and in the back of the mind, there might be the question, at what location in the world was the generic drug manufactured and what elements of quality-control were applied?

Back to the internet and to the website of GoodRx, continuing to feel short-of-breath, a scanning of available information by the patient provided remarkable news. The *generic* form of the drug would cost between $12.50 at Costco to $16.90 at CVS and *no insurance was even needed*—the patient just needed to bring the coupon printed from GoodRx and this highly-affordable 1-month supply would be available. And then, the patient remembered the insurance policy and how the monthly premium charge was up to date to stay properly insured.

Back to the computer, the insurance company's drug costs popped up on the screen: for a 30-day supply of the brand name (which they had already told him they would not cover), the cost was $208, again at Costco. For a 30-day supply of the generic drug, the cost *with insurance coverage* was $20, also at Costco.

The patient briefly wondered why, at the *same pharmacy*, for the *same drug,* the purchase of the generic drug was $12.50 *without* insurance, and yet the purchase of the same identical generic drug at the same pharmacy *with* insurance was $20! Why should the drug cost *more* with medical insurance? The patient, becoming even shorter-of-breath quickly printed the free coupon from the internet site for the generic Lanoxin, and rushed to the pharmacy for the $12.50 generic drug, briefly wondering what had happened to competition among pharmacies and was there anyone who actually cared about lowering the costs of drugs in America?

It is clear that drug prices to patients are affected by such variables including individual pharmacies, generic versus brand-name drugs, and insurance policies, but there is more! Looking at the three giant drug wholesalers of AmerisourceBergen, Cardinal, and McKesson, the Pharmacy Benefit Management (PBM), the DIR fee, coupons from internet sources like PBM-controlled GoodRx, coverage by Medicare or Medicaid, computer-generated coverage by PBM controlled OptumRx in concert with United Healthcare, how is any patient able to shop for his or her needed drugs without becoming overwhelmingly confused and likely paying too much? What is an elderly patient such as my father supposed to do? And when there are 20,000 prescription drugs being distributed throughout America, where are the sources of comparative data to allow pricing information to become easily available to the individual needing medication? This extraordinary gross obscuration of prices by the array of variables has become almost an art form in America, involving all of the entities together seeming to say, effectively, "The less you know, the better, we'll take care of the cost." This, of course, relieves them of the direct competitive price information that would drive customers away—a simple process of obscuring the price data while increasing the costs and profits.

It is noteworthy that Lanoxin, Digoxin, and all drugs in this group are "biological" drugs since they come from a plant. The drugs of Hippocrates' time were all biologic also, including charred hemp, opium, and all of the various herbs that could be ingested from plants. The molecular basis of drugs was not known in those days and the plants evolved into drugs for humans based on trial and error or effects noted by various people randomly ingesting the plants. There are many other biologic drugs used today, one of the most common being insulin, and the FDA has more recently (in 2020) redefined the term "biologic" to mean a protein that has not been chemically synthesized. The new definition further defines "protein" as any "alpha amino acid polymer with a specific sequence that is greater than 40 amino acids" truly a mouthful in any language. Under this new definition, however, insulin became considered a biological product...the purpose of this was to facilitate greater competition in the marketplace. And this competition process seems to be evolving; one of the more common insulin preparations, Lantus, currently costs $425 for five injections according to the manufacturer Sanofi; a "biosimilar" insulin, Semglee, was manufactured by Viatris and Blocon Biologics last year, and in July of 2021, the FDA declared the drug to be interchangeable with Lantus. This will now result in new competition for Sanofi, challenging their insulin costs--the cost for Semglee's five injection pens was $148 last year. Remarkably, doctors would have to *specifically prescribe* the biosimilar version, rather than allowing pharmacists to substitute it for Lantus when filling the prescription; it is hopefully presumed that medical doctors would move to the less expensive and biosimilar Semglee (since most pharmacists are not likely to call physicians to advise about the cheaper form of insulin).

The giant drug wholesalers AmerisourceBergen, Cardinal, and McKesson are the biggest in the country. If there are any doubts about how much money is involved with just these three wholesalers, it is instructive to know their annual revenue is currently about $500 *Billion per year,*[84] and continuing to increase as they are estimated to represent 90% to 95% of the wholesale drug distribution market. Why is this significant? Following the money pathway from the pharmaceutical (who face no controls over what they can charge), when these wholesalers gather and distribute these drugs to pharmacies, they typically *automatically* increase the cost by 20%.[85] These wholesalers also look at the prices charged by the pharmaceutical companies who may sell the drug directly to pharmacies, and then adjust their charges accordingly to this direct price—all of this is largely moved up and down based on *what the market will bear.*

Sick patients, like my suffering father, represent "the market," and what he can pay is continuously changing with the determination of who pays for the drug other than and beyond the patient. And so, what insurance companies might pay, or what the government would pay with Medicare or Medicaid payments can directly and immediately affect what is being charged. Also, "insurance companies" are not just "insurance companies." The broad term actually refers to other branches of this pricing spider Web which includes:[86]

- "Prescription benefit managers" the so-called PBMs previously noted, like Express Scripts, CVS Health, or OptumRx
- Health Maintenance organizations (HMOs) like Kaiser Permanente or United Healthcare

- Government programs such as Medicare Part B or D, or Medicare Advantage (Part C), or Medicaid

The variables in these charges seem to be endless, easily noted by the vast variety of drug charges at the market place for patients who directly purchase prescribed drugs. This process is challenging for many sick and elderly patients who then are inclined to go to the pharmacy where they trust the pharmacist for their medications...elderly and frail patients are inclined to ask the trusted pharmacist what the cost of a drug is, and to hope for a good answer.

Furthermore, the variables creating different prices patients will have to pay for the same drug affect *all* the drugs available, not just a common one like digoxin. There are, really, seven major variables a sick patient must face:

1. Different pharmacies each with different prices for the same drug
2. Brand name drugs versus generic drugs
3. Insurance drug coverage versus minimal or no insurance
4. The availability of government support systems like Medicare or Medicaid

5. The coverage policies of government support systems
6. The controlling mandates of the wholesalers AmerisourceBergen, Cardinal, and McKesson
7. The DIR fee paid by the pharmacist
8. The PBM controllers (including GoodRx and their coupon-generating website)
9. Drugs made by American manufactures, versus drugs made in India, China, Mexico, South Korea or other countries

And so, we keep returning to DIR and PBM as *additional* factors in this unbelievably complex mosaic of entities that controls the price of drugs patients must pay.

What is a "DIR" fee that is charged to the pharmacist and how does it affect a drug's price? This charge is like a fine against the pharmacist, regularly assessed and often seemingly arbitrary, covering some of the money a Medicare Part D plan or a plan like OptumRX or GoodRx might have to pay. This fee is supposed to "offset member costs" but it acts as more of a penalty against the pharmacy for "transgressions" that are often vague or unknown. The patient standing at the pharmacy window or the payment register knows nothing about this additional fee, of course. The pharmacist knows all about it, of course, but is generally not able to change it, beyond making an effort to dispense higher numbers of generic drugs which may or may not move the pharmacy expenses in the right direction.[87]

Finally, we move to the giant on the block of drug price controls: the PBM (Pharmacy Benefit Manager). Touted by favorable websites, the PBMs are "doing the bulk of the work for over 80% of employers in the United States."[88] The flowery description further goes on to state that PBMs "are the connectors between employers, members, drug wholesalers, pharmacies, and drug companies, working to facilitate the best possible health outcomes at the best possible costs."[89] While this sounds good for the control of drug expenses, the reality appears to be somewhat different and can explain, from the law offices of litigator David Balto, the reasons behind a long string of litigation against PBMs in the United States. Mr. Balto's site defines the current PBM circumstance, before listing numerous class action cases, as follows:[90]

In just the last few years, the major PBMs (CVS Caremark, Express Scripts, OptumRx, Prime Therapeutics) have faced numerous federal or multidistrict cases over allegations of various misconduct -- stemming from clawbacks of consumer copays; fraud; misrepresentation to plans, patients, and providers; unjust enrichment through secret kickback schemes; and failure to meet ethical and safety standards. While some of these cases are ongoing many have resulted in hundreds of millions of dollars in damages to states, plans, providers and patients so far.

PBM's would appear to profit, as the "invisible middleman" at nearly every stage of the supply chain from drug maker to the patient, and are thought to be the biggest influence on the soaring price of prescriptions.[91] Many entities and individuals have debated whether PBMs should be able to "keep" the rebates they charge and receive from drug manufacturers...it seems egregious that these rebates are never publicly disclosed.[92] Even a cursory review of the internet provides a remarkable litany from pharmacists and litigators about the actions of PBMs, identifying this hidden price-controlling network as one of the main sources of financial distress to pharmacies, closely coupled with their being forced to close their "brick and mortar" stores as other drug distribution sites rise to the top of popularity. Talking with pharmacists with their struggling "brick and mortar" stores, they easily (and angrily) provide numerous pricing labels they must attach to these patient's vials of drugs, typically: Cost of drug: $15.82, Allowed price of drug: $0.98, Patient copay: $.98, Net Charge: $0.98, Insurance Pays: $0.00. Translated, the pharmacist is charged nearly $16.00 and the patient pays *less than a dollar*. You do not need to be an economist to understand that this is leading to more and more closures of private pharmacies.

With those considerations, mixing with the thousands of prescription drugs that may be purchased in the United States, the result is a massive amount of different prices for all drugs, as hidden clusters of entities profit as they control drug distribution, while virtually none of the price alteration information is easily available to the general public.

You might ask how the drug companies, the pharmaceuticals that make the drugs, can even further inflate prices for patients needing drugs for some of the more common conditions like hypertension, diabetes, asthma, or high cholesterol. Simple! The companies effectively move doctors into the company's sphere of influence by providing those who actually write the prescriptions with *free samples of the drug* for their offices. Then, when the doctor writes for any drug for a patient's disease, he or she will think, "I'll give the patient samples, lowering the cost for the patient!"

This pharmaceutical influence on doctor prescribing can be illegal, including a recent case where a drug company's executives pushed company representatives to promote certain narcotic drug sales in predominantly rural counties across the United States. They used specific tactics like showing up at medical offices early in the morning, before the offices were even open, to reach doctors before they saw their first patient and to hype up their products while offering free trials and samples. In 2019, this activity resulted in a federal jury finding top executives of the opioid manufacturer Insys Therapeutics guilty of racketeering related to the opioid epidemic.[93]

Regarding what physicians are then prescribing, a clinical professor of orthopedic surgery at the University of California, Irvine, Dr. Charles Rosen (who is one of the co-founders of the Association for Medical Ethics[94]), testified before Congress and noted that "90 percent of medical professionals want to do the right thing and hold true to the Hippocratic Oath." He underscored this by adding that if physicians treat patients because of financial or other pharmaceutical company incentives for specific drug prescriptions, "they're breaking the oath they took when they graduated from medical school."

This creates a shadow on the common (and ethical) process of the drug company supplying "pharmaceutical reps" to help explain to the doctor how newer or more expensive drugs can work. These "reps" are loquacious, physically attractive/beautiful, engaging, and very smooth as they often bring lunches for the doctor along with drug information and more, always more and more samples. The doctor may be invited to "Drug Rep" lunches or dinners at fine restaurants for further lectures by physicians about drug mechanisms and (always subtly) the specific drugs the company is promoting. From the doctor's perspective, it all seems so nice: an attractive and pleasant rep arrives with lunch and or dinner invitation, he or she brings drug information *and samples* and regularly, an hour of engaging talk and fulfilling lunch later, the doctor's sample closet is filled with the more expensive drug. And then, potentially, there is a dinner to look forward to.

An example of this sample process is a steroid inhaler for breathing problems. A patient who needs steroid inhalation to improve airway function could take an expensive inhaler or perhaps might take one of the other drugs like the following:

- beclomethasone (Qvar)
- budesonide (Pulmicort)
- budesonide/formoterol (Symbicort) – a combination of a steroid plus a long-acting bronchodilator drug
- ciclesonide (Alvesco)
- fluticasone (Flovent HFA)
- fluticasone propionate (Flovent Diskus)
- fluticasone furoate (Arnuity Ellipta)

- fluticasone propionate/salmeterol (Advair Diskus) — a combination of a steroid plus a long-acting bronchodilator
- fluticasone furoate and vilanterol trifenatate (Breo Ellipta)
- fluticasone furoate/umeclidinium/vilanterol (Trelegy Ellipta) — a combination of a steroid, an anticholinergic, and a long-acting bronchodilator drug
- mometasone furoate (Asmanex)
- mometasone/formoterol (Dulera) — a combination of a steroid plus a long-acting bronchodilator drug

A quick price comparison analysis of brand-name steroid inhalants would be worthwhile since some inhalers contain the exactly the same corticosteroid, called fluticasone, and others contain a long-acting beta agonist (LABA) airway opener, the effects of which can last many hours. A comparison reveals that with a GoodRx internet coupon, Advair Diskus costs about $100, or $47 through the UnitedHealthcare insurance-linked Optum-Rx (for a one month supply), while brand-name Breo costs $378.94

exactly in all 10 pharmacies available. There is no competitive pricing, the Breo costs are all fixed prices at all pharmacies. While this would make most compassionate doctors want to prescribe the less expensive Advair Diskus form of inhaled steroid for their patients, what if the doctor had *samples*, lots of samples, of a more expensive steroid inhalant? The patient would be happy leaving the doctor's office with a bag of the inhaled steroid "free" samples (that would cost almost 4 times as much as the less expensive drug) and when refill time arrives, this more expensive drug would usually be requested and purchased.

It can quickly become more complicated when other common conditions like hypertension (high blood pressure) is considered. This condition may be treated by any of the following 11 *classes* of drugs, each class having several drugs within.

Diuretics

Beta-blockers

ACE inhibitors

Angiotensin II receptor blockers

Calcium channel blockers

Alpha blockers

Alpha-2 Receptor Agonists

Combined alpha and beta-blockers

Central agonists

Peripheral adrenergic inhibitors

Vasodilators

Add up all the drugs for hypertension and then try to do price comparison for the nearly 100 possible drugs—the entire process is quickly overwhelming, especially when the price of drugs is substantially affected by the multiple pricing variables, mixing with "free" samples, and the confounding forces as we have seen.

Furthermore, the digoxin and inhaled steroid examples are just some of the more common of the thousands of drugs now available—pricing data becomes even more obscure when a drug is not as readily available as these common medications. Drugs for treatment of rare conditions, or newer drugs for common conditions, are examples of this. This, more recently, might include Aduhelm that recently received FDA approval for early Alzheimer's disease—the manufacturing company, Biogen, estimates the cost to each patient needing this drug will be about $56,000 per year.[95] And, unfortunately, that cost comes only after expensive brain MRI studies and other brain tests to confirm the diagnostic criteria for the drug. Much of the expense is, of course, justified by the company in consideration of what they define as immense research costs, especially (in this case) when so many Alzheimer drugs have failed to show any benefit, and considering the expensive mysteries of researching a brain disease, the cause of which is not fully understood.

The high cost of drugs becomes particularly relevant when *new* drugs are developed, such as Pfizer or Johnson and Johnson creating their vaccines against the Covid virus. Just to develop a drug stimulating immune antibody defenses systems against a "spike protein" of a virus (seen with electron microscopy) is one of the most remarkable scientific evolutions since Hippocrates, a time when even the existence of such pathogens was of course not known. Price increases are also created when drugs are developed to combat highly challenging conditions such as the Biogen effort against Alzheimer's disease or many of the pharmaceutical efforts to combat the many different varieties of cancer. Finally, the biggest challenge contributing to high prices at this level relates to drug development against rare diseases such as Sarcoidosis and Sjogren's syndrome where future payments from a very small number of patients make it nearly impossible to recoup the cost of development.

Regarding the matter of drugs to immunize against the Covid virus, what is the price of the vaccine to patients? Which drug companies are involved in the effort, who prescribes the vaccine, and who decides if the vaccine is "approved and safe?" The Covid vaccine process has been the most politically controlled, FDA inhibited, distribution-havoc, website misinformed, Social Media ranting exercise in the entire history of our country. The companies involved in the vaccine production are numerous (Moderna, BioNTech/Pfizer, Johnson & Johnson, Novavax, Sinopharm/Beijing Institute, AstraZeneca/Univ. of Oxford, Sinovac, CanSino Biologics, and Inovio), of which Pfizer, J&J, and Moderna have dominated in the United States. The vaccine is paid for by the taxpayers, the rollout to the public was remarkably slow and badly managed by the government. For example, it seems impossible that at a time when 190 million people had been already vaccinated in the United States, the FDA had still not "approved" the vaccines for the population except under so-called "emergency use approval." This, of course, delayed many people from wanting to get vaccinated, since it had not been officially "FDA approved."

To make matters worse, the very professionals who would know best the vaccination needs of individual patients, were essentially locked out of the process. Doctors are not supplied with the vaccines in their office, unlike virtually every other vaccine in widespread use against other preventable diseases. While physicians apparently are not to be trusted to vaccinate their patients against Covid, CVS Pharmacy and other drug outlets eagerly signed up the population on their commercial websites. Shifting individual patient vaccination responsibility from the doctor to a pharmacist who doesn't know the patient and yet who can administer the drug without a prescription, or to a pharmacist who can *withhold* the same drug, potentially harms so many patients with a need for a booster shot as their antibody levels diminish. Those patients with asthma, emphysema, congestive heart failure and other increased-risk conditions, are then left without a chance to improve their vaccine protection since they don't meet the government-issued decree of being immunocompromised.

It is worth mentioning again that while the Food and Drug Administration regulates how new drugs are tested, marketed, and released on the market, the FDA doesn't have any price controls over medications. And, importantly, once a drug is approved by the FDA and released to patients, the drug's patent (like a copyright for the drug) will begin to run out, after which generic drugs may be produced without most of the development and research expenses. However, substantial protection is available for the patent duration, and it may take up to 20 years after the patent holder's drug is first filed with the U.S. Food and Drug Administration (FDA) before cheaper generic "copies" can be made. With that, and not surprisingly, a "work-around" this patent time limit has become established for the drug companies developing a unique new drug: pharmaceuticals are permitted to extend a patent by simply reformulating a drug – often simply changing the dosing recommendations or the mechanisms by which the drug is administered. Also, the drug company may create an "extended-release" version of their same drug as a common way to restart the patent timer for their products.

Our country's history of drugs and pharmaceutical companies never really began to develop until the Civil War—the 1860 doctors knew of John Wyeth and Eli Lilly, but the drugs available for battlefield casualties were highly limited. Also, additional laboratories serving the Union Army included Charles Pfizer and Company, Edward R. Squibb, Powers and Weightman (many years later to become Merck), Rosengarten and Sons, and John Wyeth—many of which are still prominent in the industry today.

Most of the thinking of doctors and the practice of medicine in our country during the Civil War was still adherent to the concepts from Hippocrates, relating to the restoration of balance within bodily systems, the *humoral theory* (in which black bile, yellow bile, blood, and phlegm needed balancing). Having to undergo surgery after a Civil War battle was nearly always equivalent to a pathway to death since infection was virtually always assured and there was no knowledge of "germ" theory or surgical procedural sterility. Ether and chloroform were available, however, and more than 95% of major Civil War surgeries[96] were performed under anesthesia. A common surgical disaster was the inflammable ether anesthetic igniting as fumes came in contact with operating room candles. Explosions in the operating room within tents or rudimentary wooden hospital structures were a disaster for the patient and often for the surgeon. Antibiotics were virtually unknown (since bacteria was unknown) and hospital gangrene after battle wounds to extremities (often caused by staphylococcus bacteria) carried about a 97% mortality.[97] The doctors of that time had to wait another nearly 70 years before the 1928 discovery of penicillin by Fleming in London. New "miracle" drugs like quinine were evolving, however, as was iodine, quinine, opium-containing "Dover's Powder" and highly toxic mercury-containing calomel (a laxative and fungicide) along with antimony and poisonous lead-based drugs.

Altogether, two-thirds of the approximately 660,000 deaths of soldiers during the Civil War were caused by uncontrolled infectious diseases, and epidemics played a major role in halting several major war campaigns. It has been estimated[98] that these delays, coming at a crucial point early in the war, prolonged the fighting by as much as 2 years. The spectrum of infection was horrific and conditions included pneumonia, typhus, typhoid, malaria, yellow fever, and even smallpox from the variola virus (although, remarkably, a rarely-provided vaccine for smallpox was available and had been known to be effective more than a half century before, in 1796). The primary problem centered on a fundamental lack of knowledge about infections and disease as the doctors struggled with limited medical understanding. The doctors' thinking continued to be based on the *observation of symptoms* rather than efforts to identify underlying causes. However, the eventual result of this loss of life during the Civil War was the stimulation of new research efforts that finally brought a more complete understanding about which drugs could be effective against the various disease conditions.

Although the drug-manufacturing companies (pharmaceuticals) created and produced medicines for America as we have seen, it was the pharmacy (and the pharmacists within) that distributed these drugs to the population of the expanding country. One of the first pharmacies (all of which were initially called apothecaries) was started by an Irish immigrant in 1729 when Christopher Marshall opened his doors of the Marshall Apothecary in colonial Philadelphia.[99] In those early days of the pharmacy evolution, the pharmacist (often called *chemists* or *druggists*) owned his or her own pharmacy; they consulted with patients regularly and it was routine for them to mix together chemicals (with the exception of narcotics) to treat various symptoms and ailments experienced by the suffering patients. In 1821, The Philadelphia College of Pharmacy was founded, representing the first step in developing a system of pharmaceutical practice in the United States. And, that same year, sixty-eight pharmacists signed the Constitution of the first pharmaceutical association that included a strict code of ethics that would expel anyone who "adulterated" medications.

By the 1900s, the drug-manufacturing companies began to supply pharmacists with various forms of pills such as tablets, coated pills, and gelatin capsules, although they still created many different kinds of liquids, ointments, creams, lotions, and ear drops for their patients. In fact, right up to the 1950s, the pharmacists often still prescribed the drugs they purchased from the manufacturing companies and subsequently dispensed to the patient in a manner based on the counseling and the experience they had from their training as well as from the previous years of observing drug effects and side-effects. The cost for these drugs, then, was largely determined by the pharmacist in his or her own pharmacy, and was based on the complexity of the formulation, the cost of the raw materials from the drug-manufacturing companies, and almost certainly was affected by an assessment of what the traffic would bear.

However, *what the traffic will bear* is being tested continuously as drugs became marketed directly from the pharmaceutical company to patients and the expansion of costs became increasingly accelerated. When drugs over the Web began to be accessed directly by the patient, there was no pharmacist to explain why any drug suddenly costs more, and then egregiously more, regularly reaching higher and higher levels. This accessing of the patient became more refined as pharmaceutical ads began to pop up on anybody's cell phone if the owner had initiated a website with any remote association with any specific drug. Furthermore, if any drugs had been purchased through a website like OptumRx, the patient's email site begins to receive "refill time" ad notifications from the company.

The government House Oversight Committee[100] conducted an 18 month investigation and, in September of 2020, revealed the widespread patterns of drug onerous pricing schemes. Their investigation revealed that, for example, Celgene and BristolMyers Squibb's drug Revlimid for cancer hiked their price 23 times since 2005, and Teva's multiple sclerosis drug Copaxone increased their price 27 times since 2007. Although the drug manufacturers often claim these price increases are the result of research and development, the committee found there was little to no direct relationship of these factors to these price hikes. The usual Democrat vs Republican back-and-forth emerged with the Democrat consensus being that "uninhibited pricing power has transformed America's pain into pharma's profit," according to Rep Peter Welch

(D-Vt.). The Republicans countered that the hearings were for the purpose of "vilifying and publicly shaming pharmaceutical company executives," according to Rep James Comer of Kentucky. The claims and counter-claims continued in typical government fashion, becoming highly personal when Rep. Katie Porter (D-CA) pointed out that the Celgene's CEO profits from Revlimid resulted in a $500,000 bonus to Celgene CEO Mark Alles. It was further noted that, as the company tripled the price of the drug, his $13,000,000 salary was "pegged to profits from that one drug," while the taxpayers had to pay $3.3 billion to the company for Medicare beneficiaries.

The one overall theme that emerged from the hearings was that Congress would be watching pricing mechanisms closely, especially when "particularly aggressive pricing strategies that depend on the U.S. market are divorced from underlying costs of manufacturing or development."

At the end of the long and tortuous path from drug development to the patient is the pharmacist and his or her pharmacy. The reality of drug purchasing in the United States is driven by the fact that the United States is the only country among those studied with a large uninsured population, and even Americans with insurance tend to have less protective benefits than people in other countries. Also, the fact that this country has virtually no price control strategies plays a role. Most countries in the world have centralized price negotiations or national formularies, as well as mechanisms for comparative and cost-effectiveness research to establish price ceilings. Notably, only the Veterans Administration and the Department of Defense are permitted by law to negotiate directly with drug manufacturers and they subsequently pay prices that are roughly half of those paid at retail pharmacies. Everybody else must pay whatever the drug manufacturer charges.

Through all of these evolutions, the private pharmacists continued their struggle, with their professional road becoming increasingly difficult. In 1951, everything changed in the wrong direction for pharmacists when the Durham-Humphrey Amendment to the Federal Food, Drug, and Cosmetic Act of 1938 shifted the role of pharmacists dramatically. For the first time, pharmacists were prohibited from prescribing medications for their patients and could dispense drugs *only with a physician's prescription*. Their role further became defined to that of ensuring the safety of medication the pharmacist sold to patients.[101] These pharmacists, then, became the suppliers of drugs as they received bulk quantities of pills from drug-manufacturing companies and then doled them out to the patients.

The concept of a pharmacist becoming downgraded to someone like a pill-dispensing clerk did not sit well with the profession, especially in light of the comprehensive training required to become a pharmacist. The pharmacy-training program is actually a long and arduous pathway, usually after obtaining a college degree, followed by starting the process of applying to pharmacy school for *another* four years of hard work and expense to achieve the degree as a Doctor of Pharmacy (Pharm.D.). The training is much like the medical school training for Doctors of Medicine (MD), requiring the successful completion of the four-year post-graduate professional curriculum, and must include a minimum of 1,740 hours of clinical experience for the emerging pharmacist. High grades were required during this training or the pharmacy student will be removed from the program. Successful completion of the training then allows the pharmacy student to enroll in and become licensed as an *Intern* Pharmacist, where he or she is required to work under the direct and personal supervision of a registered and licensed pharmacist.

Finally, since many states do not have reciprocity with other states, a pharmacy student who has graduated from a school in another state from where he or she would like to practice, or from a foreign country pharmacy program, must have demonstrated a practical pharmaceutical experience of 1,500 hours of dispensing medication, compounding of prescriptions, preparing pharmaceutical formulations, keeping records and regularly making reports as required by state and federal statutes to become acceptable for licensure. A license is then required in all 50 states and additional examinations must be taken to be granted licensure; all states require prospective pharmacists to pass the North American Pharmacist Licensure Exam, or NAPLEX, which tests pharmacy skills and knowledge. Forty three states and the District of Columbia also require the emerging pharmacist to pass the Multistate Pharmacy Jurisprudence Exam, or MPJE, which tests knowledge of pharmacy law. The eight states that don't require MJPEs instead require tests tailored to that state's specific pharmacy laws. Licensed pharmacists who might want to obtain a license to practice in *another* state may then generally obtain one without extensive retesting.

For a young man or woman who has finally completed years of this kind of training, it was professionally challenging to then be downgraded by Federal law to begin working essentially like a clerk. This all simmered for a while, and finally in the 1980s, the movement to expand the responsibilities of pharmacists again gathered traction. Finally, by 2003, the Medicare Prescription Drug Improvement and Modernization Act allowed pharmacists the privilege of, once again, counseling patients about prescription drugs as well as allowing them to give advice relating to over-the-counter medications. This gratifyingly expanded the pharmacist's role to again include the professional role of administering vaccines while counseling patients, and to provide other important patient care services. As recognized specialists, these pharmacists were then finally able to focus again on disease and chronic condition management, medication management, health and wellness, and any other services that could help improve the quality of life for the patients who come to their pharmacy.

However, with this improvement in professional recognition and the granting of expanded permissible activities, the *individual* pharmacist became unable to function autonomously or to remain separate from the expanding companies that dominated the drug dispensing (retail outlet) landscape. Whereas earlier pharmacists often owned their own pharmacy, the marketing of drugs and the expansion of drug distribution have greatly affected the professional lives of licensed pharmacists. This evolving change started, perhaps, with the marketing of drugs directly to the consumer by television.

The first televised ad for drugs had been made a couple of years after a job applicant, Liz Moench, asked the president of Boots Pharmaceuticals to describe the main customers. The president, John Bryer, answered, "Doctors." Ms. Moench asked, "Why isn't it the consumer?" and on May 19, 1983, the first televised ad for a pain reliever (Rufen) was broadcast *to the consumers* across the country.[102] The drug was a cheaper version of the common anti-inflammatory drug Ibuprofen, and the result was not to just create an uproar in the American Medical Association and the entire medical profession but also in the federal government and in the courts, while stimulating debates across America about the First Amendment of the Constitution. Lawyers took note too, since the glowing ads on television did not spell out potential risks, adverse effects, or any other negative consequence of taking the drug. The debate rages today, while the ads for medicine continue to proliferate on every television channel while expanding to computer internet sites, and the result is that drugs are now being aggressively marketed directly to people who take the drugs. Clusters of side effects are noted in some of the ads, presumably protecting the pharmaceutical company from lawsuits. It was a natural consequence that those being marketed would want to buy *directly* from the source of the marketing rather than to make a trip to the local pharmacy. Many of these advertisements even advised that a "doctor's prescription" could be provided directly to facilitate the delivery of the advertised drug.

It also was inevitable that the result of this marketing explosion has drastically affected the lives of pharmacists as well as patients by the millions who seek drugs from ever-expanding sources. And as the pharmacies and the pharmacists suffered, a new class of drug purveying white-coated "specialists" began to emerge in pharmacies everywhere: the Pharmacy Technician. A sense of this may be seen by the website[103] advising newly minted pharmacy technicians (who would be designated to work with pharmacists) about where they could find a "job." Opportunities rapidly began to exist *everywhere*, including the following:

1. Retail pharmacy where the technician may work in any one of virtually every region of the country, in big cities and even small towns, in Walgreens or CVS pharmacy departments, in Walmart, and in many grocery stores who increasingly have implanted pharmacies.
2. Hospital pharmacy where the technician will help prepare prescriptions and perform many administrative tasks, billing statements, and scheduling appointments, becoming a versatile

"team player" (presumably working with pharmacists?).

3. Clinic pharmacies, overseeing drug distribution to the clinic patients.
4. Home Care Pharmacies
5. Mail Order Pharmacies
6. Assisted living and long-term care pharmacies
7. Compounding pharmacies

Reporting for work in any of this myriad of job locations, the pharmacy technician would be required to perform the following activities:[104]

- Receiving and verifying the accuracy and authenticity of prescriptions
- Calculating the price of prescriptions
- Reviewing and recording patient information with their prescription in compliance with the guidelines of the General Pharmaceutical Council
- Stocking the pharmacy with inventory
- Providing instructions to educate people on the correct way to take their medicine
- Supporting the Pharmacist in the daily operation of the pharmacy

- Protecting employees and patients by adhering to infection-control protocols and policies
- Disbursing completed and confirmed prescriptions to patients
- Answering incoming calls and fielding patient questions
- Maintaining a clean and safe pharmacy by complying with regulations, rules and procedures

It would follow that upper-level managers of pharmacy companies *not* run by pharmacists might wonder how much work traditionally performed by pharmacists could be done by much less-expensive pharmacy technicians. It was not only easier for an individual to become a technician, since there is negligible training involved, but job opportunities in America were expanding and the appeal for taking this route became substantial. It also became apparent that it would be easier to hire technicians rather than pharmacists for a large portion of the drugstore's activities. It is worth noting that the median pay for technicians is just over $40,000 per year (averaging $17.50/hour in California in 2021[105]), the entry-level education is only a high school diploma or equivalent, the work experience needed is none (with on-the-job-training starting upon hiring). Since a pharmacist's salary is, in contrast, about $155,000 per year and since companies could hire almost four technicians for the same amount of salary as a pharmacist, it might seem more efficient and profitable to hire additional technicians, working under one pharmacist who could (increasingly) supervise the pharmacy technician activities.

This scenario has been considered, however, and most state regulations have been modified to prevent a larger ratio of technicians-to-professional-pharmacists. In California, for example, the maximum number of pharmacy technicians to pharmacists is 2:1 (although the California Business and Professions Code section 4115(f)(1) specifies that a pharmacy with only one pharmacist shall have no more than one pharmacy technician performing pharmacy technician functions.[106] In Texas; this ratio is, remarkably, 6:1.[107]

Increasingly, under this scenario, the pharmacists could become supervisors of technician employees rather than traditional pharmacists who are kept busy and spending most of their time discussing medications with patients and filling prescriptions. The step down into this supervisor-like role would be even easier if a large drugstore company owned an outlet (like in a grocery market or other facility), rather than a pharmacist having any direct ownership role in his or her pharmacy. Paying close attention to these costs, a viable business model would be to expand the number of pharmacies into a wide variety of settings, as pharmacists were ever-increasingly diminished into a shadow of their former selves. This would become even more successful if the company owning the pharmacy could control the costs of the high-demand drugs they distributed to the public.

And so, from pharmacists to pharmacy technicians, from stand-alone drugstores run by pharmacists to stores supplying perfumes, toys, and dog food down the aisle, the "pharmacy," drug distribution has moved from the hands of Hippocrates into an ever-expanding spectrum of huge pharmacy companies. All this happened as patients demanded medicine solutions to their medical problems, and discovered these solutions to be everywhere, from the mailbox to the computer, from the supermarket to the mail order companies, and seemingly from almost everywhere other than the corner drugstore. It should be noted in the Web reservoir of pharmaceutical supplies, it is estimated[108] there are 30,000-50,000 online pharmacies in the United States. And the brick-and-mortar drugstores have become, increasingly, replaced with physical "pharmacy equivalents" in the corners of various commercial stores now blanketing the country.

How much has this pharmaceutical expansion evolved in this country? It is nothing short of remarkable.

A perfect example of this expansion process is found in the evolution of CVS.[109] The first CVS ("Consumer Value Stores") outlet was founded in 1963, and by 1964 had expanded to 17 stores. In 1967, CVS (which had previously just sold health and beauty products) began to incorporate pharmacy departments. In 1969, they were sold to Melville Corporation which continued the expansion, and by 1970, they had 100 stores in New England and the Northeast. More acquisitions doubled their size by 1972 and by 1974 their sales were about $100 million. The acquisitions continued, they began providing hemophilia services as they also opened into enclosed shopping malls, finally reaching $1,000,000,000 in sales by 1985 in concert with Baxter's division's Caremark. By 1988, they expanded into home care services, and mail service pharmacy services, expanding to $1.6 billion in sales and owning 750 stores. Another 500 stores were purchased in 1990, Caremark became independent from Baxter, and under CVS, developed its own formulary of drugs, with Pharmacare emerging to provide a wide range of pharmaceutical services for employers and insurers. The enlargements continued and by 1997 and 1998, another 2,700 stores were acquired from Revco and Arbor Drugs...by 1999, CVS owned 4,100 stores in 24 states, as they also launched online prescription refills services under its Caremark system. Growth continued into Southern California and by 2005, another 700 stand-alone Sav-On and Osco drugstores were acquired from Albertsons. By 2012, CVS revenue reached $100 billion, and in 2015, they acquired Target's 1,600 pharmacies and clinics...by 2020, the company's revenue was $270 billion.[110]

Other pharmacy stores followed this lucrative pathway of expansion. Remarkably, by 2020, only three drugstore companies (CVS, Walgreen's, and Signa) supplied greater than 50% of all drugs dispensed in the United States, with CVS contributing nearly 25% of this total. Walgreen's followed a similar acquisition and expansion as CVS when, by 2019, the company bought 1,932 Rite Aid stores, increasing their percent of the retail prescription market share to nearly 20%. With Signa and OptumRx rounding out the top four pharmacies, these entities control more than 60% of the drug prescription market. And yet, within CVS, Rite Aid and Walgreens, pharmacists are reported to be struggling with understaffed and chaotic workplaces.[111] Regulatory boards and, from interviews by The New York Times, many pharmacists have described the challenges where it has become difficult to perform their jobs safely. As these pharmacists struggle to "fill prescriptions, give flu shots, tend the drive-through, answer phones, work the register, counsel patients and call doctors and insurance companies," they are also racing to meet corporate performance metrics that they feel are unreasonable and unsafe.

However, at this point, if you were to look at the future and examine the hopes of a newly minted pharmacist who wanted to make a professional living supplying medications to patients, it would almost be like a hallucination. If he or she were to consider the concept of opening an independent pharmacy to compete with the giants of CVS, Walmart, Signa and OptumRx it would be a seemingly impossible financial endeavor. However, it is remarkable that, in spite of the competition from these drugstore chains, there are still nearly 22,000 independent pharmacies in the United States,[112] representing 35% of all retail pharmacies in the country. This is, however, much smaller than the estimated nearly 50,000 online pharmacies that are continuing to expand across our country. Also, encouragingly, the pharmacists in these independent stores are aggressively seeking greater computer efficiency, greater collaboration with independent practicing physicians, while expanding the personal elements such as vaccine administration, drug delivery, and hands-on patient care, together with other valuable human elements that are desired by so many patients.

For these pharmacists, seeking to sustain the professional element of the work he or she is doing in the brick and mortar pharmacy buildings, it is clear that there can be a significantly further expansion of the linkages with patients similar to (and even better than) what CVS and OptumRx have been able to accomplish. For example, I have never received an email from a pharmacist reminding me of the need to renew a 30-day prescription for medications near the end of the course of treatment. In the meantime, I *regularly* receive emails and Web notifications about various medications I have been taking, encouraging me to renew "with a click" the meds and to expect them in my mailbox within the next several days. As I was writing this specific element, the below notification abruptly appeared across my screen, a message from OptumRx to me via email:

Refill your home delivery medication today

Dear ROGER,

Ordering your refills is easier than ever. Access the Quick Express checkout page below to review and place your order. We'll bill your credit card on file. It's that easy.

Quick express checkout

At the very least, a pharmacist could maintain local contact with patients and a vibrant delivery system, via text messages or emails, he or she could converse with me about medications, and do it *even better than the corporations*. And, if any medications were designed to make me feel better in any way, to resolve an infection or other illness, for example, a brief note asking if the meds were helping would be easy to send and would be greatly appreciated. There would be a sense that somebody besides my family and physician actually cared about my medical welfare. Coordinating this kind of back-and-forth between the pharmacist and my physician (who ordered the drugs in the first place) would convey the sense of caring so unattainable from mass-mailing notices from internet sites controlled by large and distant drug dispersing corporations. It would seem this would be highly possible to help local pharmacists re-enter the world of providing medications to their patients and letting those patients know they actually cared about the effects of the drugs. Also, wouldn't this give the pharmacist an opportunity to discuss any potential side effects that may be related to the medications? Finally, wouldn't this bring the pharmacist back into the arena of helping patients with medicine, a goal so many of them had in their hearts when they started pharmacy school?

The human element, so critical for patient relationships, the element that was a centerpiece of Hippocrates and the providing of drugs so long ago, is at the heart of the medical care today, an element allowing pharmacists to provide the very best patient care for the people of their community. Working in concert with the physicians who write prescriptions for their patient's medicines, they could join the Hippocratic tradition that has been so vital for providing the very best of patient care.

Chapter 5

The Bill and Insanity

Several years ago, the former Nevada Senate Majority Whip and casino owner Sue Lowden was asked during a tight contest for Nevada State Senator how she would suggest patients could have some information about their potential medical bill *before* being examined and treated. The question inferred that it might be helpful for patients to know in advance what the costs for their service might be. Answering the question, she reflected on the earlier days of medicine when a patient could "bring a chicken to the doctor"[113] for payment, and she alluded to this kind of solution for patients to resolve the myriad of challenges of unexpected medical charges. That idea was immediately blasted as "one of the dumbest things from a candidate for statewide office" by her opponent, and she was mocked and ridiculed by members of the opposing political party. Never allowed to define any consideration of upfront payments to help anticipate the current challenges from often unexpected medical charges, she lost the election and moved on with her life as a business owner in Las Vegas.

What Ms. Lowden was discussing was the long-ago consideration of an *upfront* payment (a chicken in the "old days") for medical care...this is indeed similar to how many patients may have determined their charges before being treated long ago. If a chicken wasn't available, an offer to paint the doctor's house or office has been advanced as a suggestion. Or, almost anything else could be offered as payment, if money was not available. *Whatever* was offered, the concept was for the patient to know in advance the approximate cost of impending medical care and to allow the patient to make an offering that would satisfy that charge. The matter of charges and *unexpected* charges to a patient, and the quagmire of our country's current billing absurdity forced upon physicians, fuels one of the most powerful elements behind patient and doctor dissatisfaction in our medical system. And, the current system, established over recent decades by the government in concert with an ever more powerful medical insurance industry, on top of bizarre input from the World Health Organization (WHO) has evolved into a diabolical process called "medical billing," summarized as follows:

- A patient arrives at the doctor's office for care, and usually does not know what charges will be forthcoming for the upcoming examination and treatment. The patient also does not know how much of any bill he or she might be required to pay after any insurance has been billed, and potentially after Medicare has been billed following the provision of care.
- Before seeing the doctor for the appointment, the receptionist usually asks the patient, "Do you have your insurance information?" Also, the receptionist might also ask, "Are you in the Medicare or Medicaid system?"
- If the answers are satisfactory, the patient is hopefully soon sitting either in the doctor's office or at the end of an examination table.
- After the doctor's review of the patient's history and after the examination, the patient is treated and prepares to leave the office, often being requested by the doctor's billing clerk to provide a "copay" payment before departure (if the clerk hasn't already collected it "up front.") The patient pays whatever amount is requested and departs

the office, hoping insurance and Medicare will cover some or maybe the entire remaining still-unknown bill.

- A few weeks later, the patient receives a bill from the doctor in the mail, advising the following:
- An additional amount of money is now due, covering what was not paid by insurance and Medicare, and this amount must be paid in 30 days or the patient will be in default. Some of the lab charges were identified as "covered" and other lab charges were not covered. Also, the charges for the cost of the ancillary procedures such as a breathing evaluation or cryotherapy for a leg wart, and perhaps for an electrocardiogram and a visual exam, were partially paid or had been determined to be "not covered."
- The bill shows that the Medicare system and the insurance company were billed for the variety of "ICD-10" codes that were the diagnostic and procedural codes relating to the patient's exam and treatment. On closer examination, it was clear that Medicare determined several of the ICD-10 codes were for conditions that were "not covered"

to pay for the procedure or evaluation; the insurance company then *automatically* immediately also declined to cover those costs "per insurance company payment protocol."

- The patient calls the insurance company to find out why there was no coverage for the charges associated with those ICD-10 diagnoses; the insurance clerk advises it is the insurance company's "protocol," spelled out in the detailed patient agreement to not pay for whatever Medicare declines to cover. The patient is then encouraged to contact "the government" and appeal the Medicare denial decision.
- In a recent patient billing example, extracted from *tens of thousands* of similar examples, if the patient had an elevated blood sugar, he or she was likely billed for the ICD-10 billing code "83036-GZ" for an "HgbA1C," an averaging blood glucose test. On the Medicare page with a set of columns clarifying the bill, there is the question, "Service approved?" and this is answered, "No." The next column says, "The amount the provider charged was $48.41" and the next column advises, "The Medicare-Approved

amount" is $0.00. Then, for even more information, is the next column: "The Amount Medicare Paid is $0.00." Finally, in a final huge bold-print block, the patient is informed: "The Maximum You May Be Billed" is $0.00. Below this pack of messages is an advisory note, should the patient have any confusion, *"If the provider knew Medicare would not pay for this item, and didn't tell you in writing before providing it, you may be owed a refund. If you have already paid, and don't hear anything about a refund within the next 30 days, contact your provider."*

- The patient looks more closely at the other charges in the bill and discovers that the medical charges that *were* covered by Medicare were actually only *partially* paid, while the insurance company paid an additional bit more.

And so it goes on and on and on, with the patient never really able to understand what the ICD-10 system is, what an HgbA1C test was, why the trusted doctor got zero payment for some things, and why only partial payment was made for the other charges. Also, the patient struggles to understand what part of the examination itself was (or was not) covered and why only a non-defined and variable percent of the charges were covered by Medicare. The one thing the patient understands with certainty is that if he or she does not pay what the bill's bottom line states within 30 days, there will be an extra "overdue payment" charge added to the bill and it will be likely that the doctor's scheduling clerk will be inclined not to schedule a future visit.

This example is representative of one bill for one doctor visit. As an experiment at some future date, it would be interesting to look at the charges from a week or two *in the hospital* and then to try and sort out what each charge was for and why some of the charges were partially paid, some were not paid at all, and many others were for items that were fully incomprehensible. Spend enough time looking at a bill like that and a psychiatrist might be needed (and the psychiatrist's bill would likely not be covered).

It becomes rapidly clear that the entire spectrum of the American medical billing system has developed into something nearly impossible for most patients to understand. It is a system of multiple cloudy layers that challenges everyone including the billing clerks. It is a system that pits patients against doctors, patients against insurance companies, doctors against insurance companies, and doctors *and patients* against Medicare.

The Medicare system provides a massive, multipage, EOMB (Explanation of Medical Benefits) which is an incomprehensible collection of legal verbiage that still leaves the patient with the same questions about non-payment. Finally, it often appears to the patient that the insurance system participants (like Blue Cross, Blue Shield, Anthem, and a truck-load of others), have become a behemoth monstrosity of billing complexity that seem to be colluding with Medicare on billing issues. At the same time, any thoughtful patient would finally understand that these insurance carriers have been able to create a system in which patients must pay, every month, ever-increasing premiums for the insurance coverage while they also create the curse of trying to understand the impenetrable explanations when the medical bill arrives. Furthermore, at the same time, (since only a percent of the doctor's submitted bill will be paid by the government and by insurance), the doctors would be logically inclined to increase their charges for each element of future evaluation and treatment, hoping the ever-declining payments from these sources will help cover at least the doctor's clerical costs as he or she repeatedly is forced to challenge Medicare and the insurance companies. Also, since the doctor often cannot find out if he or she will even be paid by either Medicare or insurance, and since Medicare often declines *any* payment, there is an additional inclination and motivation to "up-code" the ICD-10 billing system to try and get whatever payment may be granted, perhaps with a more complex code, as the denial of payments continue.

Finally, working against both the patient and the doctor, there is no information made available to the physician that indicates what diagnosis allows which procedure to be covered by what payment and, without that knowledge, the doctor must just guess what diagnosis might allow any payment for anything. The doctor makes a guess, he or she submits a charge to the patient, to Medicare and to the insurance company, and then stands by (often for months) to see what and if anybody might be inclined to pay something, *anything*. If the charge is denied by Medicare (and, of course, then *always* denied by the insurance company), the doctor is often asked to modify/alter/change/adjust the diagnosis and resubmit the bill again to the patient, who by then is usually totally confused, and also again to Medicare and the insurance company. And then, the doctor waits, and the patient also waits to see if Medicare and/or the insurance company accepts or denies payment for the bill; it has become a business of irrational absurdity.

If the patient is frustrated by all this, one might wonder how much time the doctor spends on paperwork to accomplish the billing with the hopes there would be something in return, like maybe adequate reimbursement. The doctor may think back and wonder if this billing challenge had ever been covered in medical school. An overloaded primary care physician, who works each day to schedule increasing numbers of patients with urgent needs, who must return emergency calls from patients (like a call from an elderly man in a remote desert community who can't breathe), and who must answer calls from other physicians, must then divert his or her energy to labor over ever-increasing amounts of paperwork for billing and administration. And this doctor, who then tries to *actually practice medicine and take care of people*, can easily develop something widely known as "physician burn-out."

The statistics tell the story for the billing monstrosity of primary care. Nationally, the primary care internist is ranked at almost the ***top*** of the paperwork load, compared with twenty-five other specialties, and was found to have to perform a staggering 18.5 hours per week with billing and other paperwork issues.[114] That's 18.5 hours, that could be spent helping patients, diverted to matters of paperwork. The smallest amount of time for paperwork by *other* (non-primary care) doctors is 9.8 hours, spent by ophthalmologists, and 13.2 hours spent by dermatologists.[115]

This requirement to spend nearly 20 hours per week grinding through paperwork might seem potentially rewarding, if the coding mechanisms were successful until you look at the financial reward with all this paperwork. The internist is near the bottom of the national list for successful billing reimbursement, #24 down, while ophthalmologists and dermatologists are near the top.[116] Why should so much time be wasted on paperwork as the struggle to determine the correct billing codes for services continues, along with the added burden of appealing the volumes of denials and non-payments, all while trying to take care of patients and (perhaps) even make house calls or see the patients in the hospital?

The only bright spot in this whole debacle is that internal medicine physicians have a very small percent (15%) of their submitted billings *completely rejected* by insurance companies or Medicare...possibly, all that paperwork time does result in more accurate billing? On the other hand, it is worthwhile to note the percent of internal medicine doctors who would choose their specialty again, if they had to do it all over again—was at the very bottom of the list at 66%. This compares with the ophthalmologists and dermatologists, where 95% said they would choose the same specialty again.[117]

The biggest complaint from the largest number of internal medicine doctors is the crushing burden from the maze of rules and regulations, combined with the challenges of receiving a fair reimbursement; almost 40%

of doctors listed these factors as their biggest challenge in their medical careers.[118] It seems remarkable that these doctors who are challenged by the complex symptoms and diseases in their patients would find the "biggest challenge" is digging through the maze of billing nonsense rather than going to battle with the forces of nature that might be trying to kill their patients.

But, looking at the national picture, how much of America's healthcare costs are actually spent on primary care? The payment of a chicken might cover the doctor's interview and examination, but what else is consuming so much money in this primary care arena that might seem relatively inexpensive? During this past year, the Journal of the AMA published a study[119] that analyzed where money is going and how much more money is spent for patient medical care during the past decade or so. The "cost of physicians' services" ranked #2 on the list (just below #1, hospital care), and was measured at 15.6% of the total healthcare costs, while all the remaining packets of categories were a smaller percentage. Furthermore, the cost of this care has been skyrocketing over the past decades (as a percent of our Gross Domestic Product), rising from 7% in 1970 by a whopping 18% in 2016, an increase of more than 2 ½ times from earlier years. The "physician care part" is worth exploring since the greatest increase in costs were for the following conditions:

- Low-back and neck pain: $57.2 billion
- High blood pressure: $46.6 billion
- High cholesterol: $41.9 billion
- Depression: $30.8 billion
- Urinary disease: $30.2 billion
- Osteoarthritis: $29.9 billion
- Bloodstream infection: $26 billion
- Falls: $26 billion
- Oral disease: $25.3 billion

A careful look at these conditions, costing everybody in the country more than $300 *billion* per year, suggests that almost all of these conditions could be cared for by a well-trained *and available* primary care doctor in a manner that should cost less, a great deal less. But, considering the billing challenges, how much do fearful patients delay their care by the threat of having to pay the increasing costs for primary care, and how much preventable disease may worsen because of this fear? A recent study[120] has suggested that 44% of Americans refused to go to a doctor because of their fear of high costs, and nearly half of those surveyed decided to skip a test or a treatment because of these costs. Perhaps not too surprisingly, it was also noted that many of those patients who avoided treatment *actually had medical insurance*. Although the question was not asked, it would seem likely that the morass of this mysterious ICD-10 billing system would play a role in the fear patients have (with or without insurance) of receiving incomprehensible bills that demand payment, quickly followed a few weeks later by red-marked envelopes from collection companies.

For a patient looking for a reasonable charge for medical care, the insanity of charges, reimbursement, and billings rages across the entire medical system in a manner that defies any element of common sense. A simple frequent example of this would be the experience of a woman in our own community looking to have her annual screening mammogram performed by her local radiology center. She is sent by her primary care doctor (if she has been able to find one) for this crucial study that may protect her from the potential of having an advancing breast cancer. She walks into the center and before proceeding with the study, she decides to ask what the charge will be for the study. It is a simple question, she would simply like to know what the mammogram is going to cost before proceeding. The receptionist has no clue as to what the answer might be and so she is sent to the billing department where the billing clerk indicates the cost is determined by "many variables." The patient points out that she would like to proceed without variables...just a standard mammogram so she doesn't have to worry about breast cancer. And so, she asks again, what will the cost be? The billing department clerk refers her to the *manager* of the billing department who sits the patient down in a private office and asks, "Do you have insurance...and furthermore, are you in the Medicare system...also, do you have Medicaid coverage...or are you trying to pay for all of this by yourself today or within the next 30 days?"

The patient answers the questions but asks again, what is the charge for the mammogram *irrespective of what insurance or government program might be available*?

The manager explains:

- The charge for the mammogram is generally between $1,000 and $1200.
- However, if she is in the Medicaid system, the payment for the study will be 100% of what is allowed, "free" as far as the patient is concerned, although the radiologists will be collecting about $200. Unspoken is that the taxpayers will be charged for this "free" study.
- Furthermore, if she is in the Medicare system, the payment returned to the radiology center for this billing will be $230 for a 2D and 3D tomosynthesis study, although a secondary return may add 20% of what isn't covered. Also, if the woman's breasts are dense, there will be a higher charge. If only one breast is dense, and the other breast is not dense, they will pay the higher charge for only that one breast, while the charge for the other breast will be the usual charge. If a "dense breast charge" is made for a breast that is *not really that dense,* there will be no payment and considerations of billing fraud will be raised.

- Another important billing fact is that, if she does have insurance, the bill will be $169, and the radiology center expects they will collect most of that.
- However, again, if she does have insurance, whatever insurance *doesn't* pay will be her responsibility.
- Finally, if she has no insurance and she has no Medicare and no Medicaid, and if she is directly paying in cash, the charge will be $280.
- But, as a courtesy to you, she is told, if you wait until "Breast Awareness Month," and you have no insurance or Medicare coverage, the charge for you will be $150.

The patient notes that "Breast Cancer Awareness Month" for that radiology center is seven months away and her primary care doctor has told her she needs the mammogram *now*. She is advised again by the billing manager that "Breast Cancer Awareness Month" is still seven months away no matter *when* she needs it. The patient knows, without asking, that although she already possesses an excellent "breast cancer awareness" of the risks of breast cancer, she will still have to wait seven months to obtain the lower charges; she would have to wait until the time arrives that is defined as the radiology company's "awareness" month. If the patient finally asks if these charges for the mammogram are posted anywhere in the facility or online, so she can compare charges with other facilities, she is told "there are too many variables and too complicated" to post anywhere.

It is the reality in today's world of assorted "coverage" systems that those companies trying to provide quality radiology services, lab services, pathology services, surgical services, and every kind of other medical service will often charge as much as 10x more for patients with insurance or Medicare coverage. In trying to conduct their business, these companies find that about 20% of all billings are immediately rejected by the systems, returning the overworked billing specialists to their vast collection of ICD-10 diagnosis codes to renew a billing in a manner that might allow for a payment. Hospital administrators will deal with the payment shortages in different ways, and in some facilities, occasionally and egregiously, these financial managers enter the hospital room of a patient recovering from surgery and, knowing this particular patient is financially wealthy, will actually ask about the possibility of future donations or sponsorships to improve the facility's bottom line. This kind of solicitation, while not being illegal, seems almost outrageous but it has been reported by aggrieved patients after finally getting discharged from more disreputable facilities.

It is worth looking more closely at what exactly this ICD-10 system is that seems to create confusion and which appears to control everything for the patients and doctors in the massive industry of medical billing. A nice-sounding answer to any question relating to ICD-10 comes directly from Medicare: *ICD-10 is the standard transaction code set for diagnostic purposes under the Health Insurance Portability and Accountability Act (HIPAA). It is used to track health care statistics/disease burden, quality outcomes, mortality statistics and billing.*[121] Unfortunately for those patients who might be called upon to actually pay for medical services, the coding mechanism is also used to determine what is allowed to be paid and how much the insurance industry will or will not pay using criteria that is not easily identified by the public. It is a secret process, and nobody can just look on an internet website to see how much the government would allow for various codes

A quick look at the "CMS" (Centers for Medicare and Medicaid Services) site, where the billing originates, may help further the appreciation for the gigantic labyrinthine the ICD-10 represents. This government site (located at www.cms.gov/icd10) is a classic government information area that obfuscates and confuses even the most diligent student of the billing system (significantly, including patients and physicians, and likely most readers of this book). A typical information blurb from this site helps illustrate the relatively incomprehensible information that is used by insurance companies and government accountants who work in various large billing-clerk loaded buildings scattered around the United States follows:

ICD-10 Implementation Date: October 1, 2015. Code services must be provided on or after Oct 1, 2015 with ICD-10; this includes Code services provided before Oct 1, 2015 with ICD-9, even if you submit the claim after Oct 1, 2015, and the ICD-10 transition is a mandate that

applies to all parties covered by HIPAA, not just providers who bill Medicare or Medicaid. About Code Sets: Code sets classify medical: Diagnoses, Procedures, Diagnostic tests, Treatments, Equipment and supplies, and they inform diverse health care functions, from billing to tracking public health. HIPAA Code Sets: Code sets outlined in HIPAA regulations include: ICD-10 – International Classification of Diseases, 10th edition, Health Care Common Procedure Coding System (HCPCS), CPT-Current Procedure Terminology, CDT – Code on Dental Procedures and Nomenclature, and NDC – National Drug Codes

Primary care doctors across the United States who might consider seeking a chicken for payment, even a tiny chicken, and any rural physicians who might *not* have a high-speed computer with ICD-10 references might just as well surrender their medical license...initiating accurate billing, or actually providing *any* billing to the government in this system is almost impossible. In the offices where a wide spectrum of primary care is delivered, the doctors who try to be successful as they struggle with this system must first hire a team of coding specialists to guide what should be charged for the various conditions found among the patients in the practice.

You might then also want to ask, why is it ICD-***<u>10</u>*** and not ICD-9, or 8, or maybe ICD-2 or 3? How long did it take to get all the way up to 10 from the bottom? You also may wonder, since this seems to be a system that is rapidly moving out of control, is it expanding exponentially to approach the very limit of technology's microchip memory capabilities? The answer is, unfortunately, yes.

A brief history may be rewarding: It all started when England passed the Registration Act in 1837 with provisions to gather more information about deceased populations and various causes of death. Eventually, ICD-1 was created before WW1, in 1909, and languished until after WW2 when, in 1946, the United Nations delegated responsibility for coding to the World Health Organization (WHO).[122] As medical knowledge advanced, it became clear that ICD-1 was grossly inadequate, and additional codes rapidly began to be added. ICD-1 advanced to ICD-2, with a few more codes, and then ICD-3, and 4, and a little more than 20 years later, ICD-8 had gone into effect, but then, within a year, ICD-9 arrived and became formalized in 1979 to be eventually used in the United States. Nothing much else happened until ICD-10 arrived and was adopted in 1990 by the WHO; however, noting the continuous and rapid evolution of diagnoses, the United States delayed implementation for about 25 years while they "studied the details of the matter."

Various countries around the world (including the United States for mortality purposes) then finally used the ICD-10 coding system and, in 2002 it was published in 42 languages but still not adopted by the United States, as we continued to "study the details." In the year 2008, it was decided that ICD-10 could actually be used in this country but then nearly another decade passed before the details had been adequately studied and it finally was implemented in October, 2015. Amazingly, three years ago, the WHO established that ICD-11 was going to be released and so now the United States will wait for another decade or two, studying the details, before the array of new codes will descend upon us.

The "details" are impressive. How many codes are covered by this ever-expanding category system that doctors must dig through to find the proper billing numbers? As noted in the latest expansion up to 2015, ICD-9 had identified 3,800 procedure codes that would hopefully take care of identifying most procedures. However, in the final 2015 release, it was apparent that there had previously been not *nearly* enough codes, and with the implementation of ICD-10, the 3,800 procedures expanded to more than 70,000 procedure codes! Furthermore, the number of *diagnosis* codes (which had been set at 14,000 prior to 2015) climbed to more than 69,000 codes.

And so, *it has actually been determined by the WHO and our government that there are 69,000 separate diagnoses to be considered while taking care of patients.* This information is generally concealed from students during medical training--if medical students knew that they needed to establish one of 69,000 possible diagnoses while studying in their anatomy or pathology class, some of them would have either started taking antidepressants or simply left medical school to seek another career pathway. Finally, with this volume of human suffering all coded so thoroughly, the patient must always remember that if the doctor's bill is not paid adequately by the government or by the insurance company, the patient always has the right to appeal (and the doctor can then presumably come up with a different code, a *better* code, *a more relevant* code, a code that yields more money) unless the patient becomes too sick during the months it took to pursue that effort.

If Sue Lowden were still running for office, a call to her suggesting she re-introduce the Chicken-for-Payment concept might receive a better reception from the voters.

And so, while there are now over 70,000 ICD-10-PC "procedure codes" telling what treatment the patient received, and over 69,000 ICD-10-CM "clinical modification" codes (known as diagnosis codes) telling the reason for seeking the doctor's care, it would seem possible that the doctor can finally just pick and choose the code for whatever procedure or diagnosis seems appropriate and that should work. It would seem so...but it is not so. Even with 69,000 diagnosis codes available for the doctor to choose (pending, of course, the upcoming ICD-11), there are unending pitfalls that will snarl even the most diligent primary care doctor trying to do the right thing.

First, what conditions are covered by ICD-10? Just to be contrary, is there *any* human condition that a treating physician could find that is NOT covered by ICD-10? Is there *any* condition so bizarre and so out-of-the-world of normal human experience, that it just could not be found? Perhaps a condition like, perhaps, *Injuries* from something not just unusual but probably impossible...like "*Water Skis on Fire*?"

A quick review of ICD-10 reveals, yes! There is a code for injuries associated from burning water skis that have regretfully become "on fire": **V91.07XA, "Burn due to water-skis on fire, initial encounter**." The doctor must first ensure that if the patient's burns were indeed from his flaming skis, and must confirm that the event was *only* the "initial encounter." *Subsequent* burning water ski injuries would not be covered by this code; there is, in fact, no code that covers a *second* event of burns from flaming water skis, perhaps with the assumption that nobody would be likely to *twice* suffer such an injury. Finally, it is left up to the most challenged mind in the most heavily-fortified high-rise insurance complex to know, for billing purposes, what percent of the burned legs or arms (or whatever) would be reasonably covered by V91.07XA?

If billing for "injuries from flaming water skis" works, it may be worth it to try another completely impossible circumstance of human medical need, where accurate billing might be so important: What about if a patient is rushed into the doctor's medical office, bleeding from his head after a hunting expedition in the Florida swamps? After taking the medical history from the patient and his friends, it becomes clear to the doctor that the patient had recently shot a duck, flying high in the sky. The duck, dying as it fell, takes retribution on the hunter and manages to target and descend directly onto the shooter's head, knocking him out and creating a serious injury. His hunting buddies scoop the hunter up from the ground, race him to the doctor's office, and after patching him up, the doctor decides to send a bill. What code could he use? What code could he *possibly* use, to be accurate? "Trauma to the head?" "Brain contusion?" Or, maybe, "Lacerations to the Scalp" or "Hit by Foreign Object?"

No! The doctor should use the handy **ICD*-10-CM Code W61. 62* – *"Struck by duck."***

This wasn't just trauma to the hunter's head. This was, clearly, a situation of a patient being *"Struck By a Duck"*! That would be the correct code to use. Also, it is worth noting that there is no code, in the entire ICD-10 that covers, "Struck by Flaming Water Skis." Apparently, during the decades of studying details to create ICD-10, *somebody* determined that *nobody* would ever be struck by flaming water skis.

Next, somehow, in the middle of this coding morass, the government or insurance billing system will determine what per cent of the doctor's bill will be allowed to cover the injury from the water skis or the dying duck. *Then, after all that*, the insurance company, seeing that the ICD-10 system actually includes an acceptable code for these injuries, has to figure out how much it will pay the doctor for medical services for treating burned legs or a falling duck head injury. The patient, of course, will have to pay the remainder. It would have to be a low amount of reimbursement, almost guaranteed, but appeals from the doctor are often possible, and even probable if he or she has a team of ICD-10 savvy billing clerks in the office with a couple of lawyers adding their billable hours to the scenario.

And on and on it goes, as it becomes apparent that there are codes for almost (but not quite) EVERYTHING!

Another challenge is to determine how specific a code must be for fair payment. For example, if a pediatrician notes that his or her child patient is significantly below normal body weight, there would be the need for the most specific possible diagnostic code to allow payment. With 69,000 available codes, it would seem this would be easy. Furthermore, the correct code for the skinny pediatric patient could even be a legal issue from lawyers representing malnourished kids...stringent attention to the correct diagnosis code is *mandatory*.

The primary care pediatrician evaluates the huge volume of potential codes and after several hours of search, a code relating to inadequate food intake is found: ***Z59.4. Lack of adequate food and safe drinking water***. A perfect code...except for the "water" part. While the code unfortunately specifies that *lack of safe drinking water* is a part of the code, in this patient, there is no sign of dehydration. The child's water intake seems to be fine, he is just a skinny kid with a low body weight. So now, how can the doctor bill for inadequate food intake if "lack of safe drinking water" is defined to be a part of the code? Wouldn't that be billing incorrectly, potentially illegal or fraudulent? Would there be legal penalties for such an incorrect coding? Would the Environmental Protection Agency study the child's potentially contaminated water source and would the lawyers representing malnourished kids take notice of additional damages for the water issue?

A closer review is needed, and like a blessing, further clarification is offered in the guidelines section of the ICD book, where a clarification specifically refers to this code: *Regarding the code Z59.4: The word "and" should be interpreted as either "and" or "or" when it appears in a title such as the code Z59.4 "Lack of adequate food* ***and*** *safe drinking water." The doctor is thereby advised that a diagnosis of "lack of adequate food" must be coded Z59.4, despite the fact that unsafe drinking water may not be a problem.*

Easy to understand: ***The word "and" actually means "and, or or."***

So, now it all becomes clear. Also, in a future case of isolated *dehydration*, where a patient is dehydrated but has adequate food, the doctor may put down the diagnosis code Z59.4 even though the code includes "lack of adequate food." Simple, as long as the doctor recalls that the word "and" means "**and** or **or**."

How did all this happen? How did we move from a doctor visit that was for the purpose of treating a patient along the mandates of the Hippocratic Oath, to now becoming reshaped into a "provider" nightmare that requires the interaction with such a labyrinthine of a billing system that regularly results in such incomprehensible double-speak havoc?

When doctors graduated from medical school, this billing system was never mentioned prior to their solemn recitation of the Hippocratic Oath. It was never mentioned anywhere in medical training since the reason for training is to learn about and diagnose disease while learning how to treat patients, a complex requirement in itself. This ICD-10 is almost like a creature that somehow came crawling up out of a dark hole on the other side of a mysterious government swamp; this creature has now infiltrated our entire medical system and the government has told us we must use it. The system is here and now it must be used. And, it *will* be used...if you want to get paid. It will be used even though the changes in the original ICD-1, a change that has taken more than the last *century* of time, has become the current ICD-10 monstrosity that is ever more complex and more impossible to properly apply to the patient's billing. And, of course, ICD-11 is lurking right around the corner.

A further detriment of this billing system is in the removal of any semblance of competition...if nobody knows what anybody else charges with variable codes, where is there any incentive for any doctor to ever *lower* his or her charges? Also, if *both* legs are burned by the raging flames of water skis on fire, can the code be used *twice*? Would different doctors use different codes? *Everybody* has to use the correct ICD-10 for billing, and if the same code is used by different doctors, since the government and insurance companies have already set the price for the code, how can there be competition if the payment will be the same? The only difference in price would be what the doctor charges the patient, since ICD-

10 charges are fixed in this secret system known only to the government and the insurance company.

Also, lost in the debris of this creation is that, if one doctor requires an hour of his valuable and limited time to properly take care of a problem while another doctor races through in 30 minutes with less effort and less attention to detail, both doctors use the same procedure code and both doctors get *exactly the same* payment. Like so many elements that are thrust upon us from the government, the incentive to do a better job, to be more thorough, to *take better care of the patient*, is completely lost. It is left up to the doctor to be conscientious, and to do the right thing irrespective of a potential financial penalty for doing so.

There is no internet site or other information source that lists competitive charges for the patient from one doctor to another, as there is with virtually every other business activity for which we pay our money. If you want to go out and buy a tool of some kind, for example, you can look at the Costco website, the Amazon website, or the Home Depot website, and pick out the lowest price of the three. But, how do you compare competing doctor's coded charges? It is not like the charge will be a big chicken versus a smaller chicken. Also, why should any doctor even be inclined to lower the medical charges when the billing is sent to the insurance company and Medicare before the patient even receives his or her often-shocking bill? The fixed reimbursement from the "third party" payers for whatever code is used will not be changed, no matter how much the doctor charges...only the patient will have to make up the difference, Medicare permitting, when higher charges are delivered to his or her mailbox. And so, prices continue to climb, and medical care in the United States has indeed become, by far, the most expensive for patients in the world.[123] The shocking differential cost for medical care is (in 2019, per capita) $10, 586 in the United States, $5,986 in (second-highest) Germany, and $4,070 for the United Kingdom and a bit more for Canada.[124]

Regarding expensive medical care, as an experiment, try asking the insurance industry: Why is our medical care so expensive? If you should ask the Blue Cross Blue Shield Association, here is their online confusing answer:

The price of medical care is the single biggest factor behind U.S. healthcare costs, accounting for 90% of spending. These expenditures reflect the cost of caring for those with chronic or long-term medical conditions, an aging population and the increased cost of new medicines, procedures and technologies.[125]

So, now we understand. As the insurance industry has explained, we have (uniquely in America) a country with an "aging population." We have patients with chronic and long-term medical conditions. Also, new medicines cost more money. Finally, we have procedures and technologies. Since Blue Cross Blue Shield Association implies that since other countries must *not* have these kinds of issues, since they are vastly less expensive, how have they helped us understand why our medical care is "the most expensive in the world"? Now, we can begin to understand why insurance premiums keep climbing to levels that would have been unbelievable just a few years ago although the new Price Transparency Rule the government is working to initiate is a step in the right direction.

Another consideration, perhaps to help lower costs, would be for the doctor to set up a quasi-clinic called an HMO (Health Maintenance Organization), like Kaiser Permanente or, alternatively for some Medicare patients, an ACO (Accountable Care Organization). The Kaiser information sources[126] indicate that Kaiser Permanente is an "HMO plan with a Medicare contract." Enrollment in Kaiser Permanente depends on contract renewal, and you must reside in the Kaiser Permanente Medicare health plan service area in which you enroll. This concept involves *groups* of doctors, hospitals, and other "health care providers," who come together "voluntarily to give coordinated high-quality care" to their patients. ("Voluntarily" and "High-Quality" contrasting with coerced and low-quality, which by implication needs to be avoided?) It is explained that, in Medicare's traditional fee-for-service payment system, doctors and hospitals generally are paid for each test and procedure they order. That drives up costs, by rewarding "providers" for doing more, even when it may not be needed.

ACOs don't do away with fee for service, but they create an incentive to be "more efficient" by offering bonuses when "providers" keep costs down.[127] The ACO makes "providers" jointly accountable for the health of their patients, and tries to accomplish this by laying out a long list of "financial incentives" to allow those "providers" to "cooperate and save money by avoiding *unnecessary* tests and procedures."[128] In fact, they make the remarkable claim that the "providers" will actually *make money* by ***not*** doing "unnecessary" tests; what is necessary and what is unnecessary will be defined by the "provider" who, under this system, makes more money by *not* doing tests. The political elements of this concept is noted at the Kaiser Healthnews website during the Obama administration: "*ACOs have become one of the most talked about new ideas in Obamacare*." For each patient in this system, doctors (or, as the ACO repeatedly says, "Providers") have a choice during the provision of care: do more tests to nail a complex diagnoses and the doctor's "bonus" is reduced. Do fewer tests, or maybe do *no* tests, and the doctor gets a bigger bonus, rewarding the doctor for doing *nothing for the patient*. This is a good thing, under ACO provisions, especially if the diagnosis is uncertain? An extension of that consideration would be if your car with a rough-running engine needs to be fixed with this kind of system for payment, you would tell the mechanic you will pay him *more* if he does *less*...and then see how well your car runs when he is finished?

There was no mentioned incentive in any ACO information source of one of the primary provisions of medical care morality as defined in the UCLA Hippocratic oath:

To the best of my ability and judgment I will practice the Art only for the benefit of my patients. The Hippocratic Oath does NOT say, I will ***not*** practice the Art for the benefit of receiving a higher bonus. In the meantime, 31% of doctors in this country participate in an ACO, and in California, nearly two thirds of doctors are taking care of patients within an ACO.[129]

Note the widely-utilized word "provider," a term that is universal throughout the ACO system. A "provider" implies a physician or medical doctor, and it sounds nice. What could be bad about somebody who "provides?"

In fact, a "provider" does not necessarily have to have completed even a single semester of medical school. To be a "provider," does one even have to graduate from high school? The actual synonyms of a provider, [130] include: "A person or thing that provides something" and furthermore may be any of the following individuals: a supplier, a donor, a giver, a source, a contributor, a benefactor, a mainstay, followed by *fifty other* "provider" definitions including a "lady bountiful" and a "fairy godmother." Clearly, a "provider" may be almost anything or anybody, as the ACO may be ready to pay for doing less.

Why is this ubiquitous term "provider" used by ACOs and others controlling doctors' medical services? In the Orwellian world of medical double-speak, the term "provider" is used since it implies to patients that the healthcare company is referring to medical doctors. They are not, specifically, but it *sounds* like they are. And, although they may, or may not, be referring to physicians, the term "provider" gives an impression that a healthcare entity has many more doctors than actually may exist within the organization. As we have seen, to an ACO, a "provider" *may* be a doctor of medicine or osteopathy, but within the walls of the medical company, he or she may also be a podiatrist, or a dentist, a chiropractor, a clinical psychologist, an optometrist, a Nurse Practitioner, a nurse-midwife, or a clinical social worker, or finally, a provider may even be a Christian Science practitioner.[131]

In the United States, where the Hippocratic Oath is still recited upon graduation in around 50% of medical schools, the process of practicing *"for the benefit of my patients"* has been transformed into a mutation away from this very essence of being a doctor. And, as the concept of "physician" has been replaced with the word "provider" in the United States, the Hippocratic concept has become watered down into a state of near-nonexistence.

The two most recognized "providers" in most medical systems are Physician Assistants (PAs) and Nurse Practitioners (NPs). While PAs and NPs are both considered "mid-level providers," PAs are trained in the medical model similar to physicians, and NPs are trained in the nursing model (as they are trained as nurses first). As the business managers of clinics study costs, there has been the replacement of physician medical practitioners with PAs and NPs, both of whom generate significant financial implications for the clinic: higher availability and lower cost. However, the Physician Assistant, under the guidance of the American Academy of PAs (AAPA), has worked to sustain similar Hippocratic principles that govern physicians' moral behavior; this is outlined in the organization's Guidelines for Ethical Conduct.[132]

A review of the American Association of Nurse Practitioners (AANP)'s "Standards of Practice,"[133] suggests that there is an analogous provision that creates a similar set of principles; the revered Florence Nightingale Pledge has been replaced in many schools by the International Pledge for Nurses. Those nurses entering the Nurse Practitioner profession must first graduate from nursing schools where most of them recite the following (taken from UCLA's graduating class of nurses):

In full knowledge of the obligations I am undertaking, I promise to care for the sick with all the skill and understanding I possess, without regard to race, creed, color, politics or social status, sparing no effort to conserve life, to alleviate suffering and to promote health. I will respect at all times the dignity and religious beliefs of the patients under my care, holding in confidence all personal information entrusted to me and refrain from any action which might endanger life or health. I will endeavor to keep my professional knowledge and skill at the highest level and to give loyal support and cooperation to all members of the health team. I will do my utmost to honor the international code of ethics applied to nursing and to uphold the integrity of the professional nurse.

The sustaining of these moral standards among PAs and Nurse Practitioners is encouraging although these two professions have also been affected by the billing activities of insurance and the government. Furthermore, the actual delivery of care throughout the world has become permeated with so many variables beyond the title of the "provider," so many differences in billing systems, payments, physician credentialing processes, legal liabilities, and numerical shortages of available doctors that the original mandate of Hippocrates has almost disappeared. As I have noted, in the United States, the Hippocratic Oath (or some variance of it) is still recited upon graduation in about half of medical schools, and yet the implementation of the oath's principles has been transformed by the American billing systems into a diminutive reflection of the original. And the first step was to eliminate the word "physician" and replace it with "provider."

If you are sitting in the waiting room and the receptionist announces, "The provider will see you now," you might want to review again why you were hoping a *doctor* might be taking care of you as you walk into the arena of "bonus-incentivized" variable providers who are "efficient and keeping costs down while providing high-quality services and avoiding tests."

What are the "incentives" to "keep the costs down"? More rapid visits, higher volumes of patients, fewer tests, selective referrals, limited hospital admissions, earlier hospital discharges, and limited choice of everything, from the physician to the mid-wife or to the Christian Science practitioner—this is how incentives work? Lessen the care, lessen the choice of hospitals or specialists, all in the name of creating "bonuses" for those providers who can limit their billable charges as they produce what is consistently defined by company managers as "quality care?" Does it work to lower costs? The bottom line of savings is revealed by Revcycleintelligence.com (https://revcycleintelligence.com). *There are about $314 million in net Medicare savings, with 34 percent earning shared savings payments. Also, fifty-six percent of ACOs saved compared to their benchmark, with 31 percent earning shared savings payments.*[134] Translated, as the providers reduce care, they earned extra payments for their portion of the "shared savings."

There was no comment from ACOs regarding the concepts that Hippocrates defined the basic cornerstone of decent and proper medical care. There has been considerable comment from medical doctors, who have spent hundreds of thousands of dollars and over a decade for training to be lumped together in this "shared savings" process of denial with other "providers," some of whom may have just a few months of training out of high school.

Are these doctors in these ACOs pulled into this system immediately after their medical school and residency training? More commonly, after a new primary care doctor has spent some time struggling with the billing challenges of private practice, and as he or she tries to provide the best possible medical care for the patient, that doctor might become increasingly inclined to "join a clinic" and to then be allowed to simply take care of patients while the clinic billing clerks "take care of the billing." Is it possible that "working for an ACO manager" might be easier than working *for the patient*? In fact, this migration is occurring daily. Last year, the share of physicians who changed their careers into ACO providers working as employees for other medical systems (such as Kaiser) surpassed the portion of doctors that own their practice for the first time, according to the AMA.[135] These other medical systems often include a hospital employing a whole collection of "providers," including those in a radiology unit, PTs in physical therapy, technicians in labs, and others.

This fundamental transition from a private practice to an ACO or hospital system has gutted the primary purpose of being a doctor for most physicians, the purpose for which they entered the profession of medicine: first and foremost to treat disease and to help patients. And, it is the billing of these patients (and their payer systems) that create so much pain from the substantial rise in costs and the bonus-driven declines in the quality of care. When the doctor works for an organization, he or she is pressured to coordinate the patient's care with the organization—the radiology units, the labs, the speech therapists, the colonoscopy physicians, the other specialty doctors, and these closed-shop referrals generate money for the organization, taking it from the patient and the insurance company/government. Is the best specialty doctor for referral of a patient the best specialty doctor *actually available in the community*, or is he or she just the specialty doctor who happens to be a member of the organization?

This can be egregious in the arena of cost. For example, in a recent Wall Street Journal article[136] on this subject, a hospital system of doctors earns an average of $1.8 million annually in revenue from a single internal medicine physician's admissions, (including referrals for tests and other services, plus practice revenue for the employed doctor). The same service often costs twice as much, or more, as compared with an independent doctor's office according to an analysis of dozens of medical services. Yet, these are the *same* services, presumably using the *same* ICD-10 codes, for the *same* conditions, and they cost the patient (insurance/Medicare) *twice as much as that from an independent physician*?

How, exactly, is a patient supposed to know about this doubling of charges as he or she looks at the billing and the demand for payment within the next 30 days?

And, nowhere in any readily available medical cost information source is there any side-by-side comparison to allow the patient to seek out a less expensive alternative to the referral provided by his or her doctor. The patient has to rely on the clinic/hospital employed doctor to make "appropriate referrals," that is, a referral in the patient's best interest, not in the best interest of the clinic or in the interest of a bonus return. Unfortunately, the patient is not informed of the cost differences and, in spite of it all, is still inclined to trust the referring doctor and to believe that such referrals would be in his or her best interest.

While this may be true, why is there no requirement for an employed internal medicine doctor to provide the patient with alternative, (i.e., *lower cost*, or perhaps higher quality, referrals)? The obvious answer is that the referring doctor would no longer have a job with that medical enterprise, when the $1.8 million revenue for the organization from that one physician drops to an amount that provides a patient equal and decent care at lower cost? Is that referring doctor *really* following the ethical guidelines of which Hippocrates spoke, and did that doctor actually pledge to follow the Hippocratic Oath upon graduation, or is the guidance of the doctor nothing more than a fulfillment of the directions from the employing organization?

As our country's healthcare costs continue to spiral up out of sight, isn't this something that should be addressed by our elected representatives? A step in the right direction to allow an open comparison of prices occurred in late 2020 with a so-called "Price Transparency Rule," that mandates private insurance companies must provide patients with more information about out-of-pocket charges. The action came during the final days of President Trump's administration, with the White House ordering private insurance companies to post negotiated prices for 500 "shoppable" services by 2023, subsequently extending to all services by 2024. Insurance companies have taken offense at providing this information for patients, and have criticized price comparison initiatives as "too expensive and burdensome," while pontificating that patients are "unlikely to shop around" for lower prices. This policy, however, allows patients to gain access to cost-sharing and price information, allowing them to know how much care will cost before going into treatment, according to the Department of Health and Human Services and is expected to help lower health-care costs to patients. At the time of this writing, the price transparency mandate is being litigated in a U.S. Court of Appeals as the insurance industry struggles to continue concealing cost differences from patients.

Since no resolution for this worsening medical billing process is available from insurance companies, we might change focus to the government. Also, since the government (in collaboration with the WHO) was instrumental in creating this ICD-10 billing system, and since the insurance companies subsequently jumped aboard, shouldn't our primary efforts to seek cost improvement be addressed to our elected representatives? Since they represent us, they should care, right? And also, since this is not a new issue, what do our representatives have to say about this and what can they do to improve the situation that is now creating ever-increasing barriers to finding good care at a reasonable cost?

To understand the thinking of our government representatives, it is helpful to ask about which system representatives currently use for their own medical care, what is their personal billing experience, and how is their medical services financed? Where does a House Representative, or a Senator, go for health care and how does he or she pay for it? Do they and their staff struggle with Medicare or other government billings, do they scrutinize their insurance company's billing statement? Do they have a knowledgeable staff member study the ICD-10 billing codes? No, like a Congressional surprise benefit, provided for the members of Congress immediately as they are elected (and provided to all Supreme Court Justices) is a system that would be remarkable if it were not so exclusive.

With no significant personal expense, these Members of Congress and the Supreme Court enjoy the pleasure of being cared for at the **Office of Attending Physician Services** (OAPS).

For a very low flat annual fee (set by the Senate at $520 and by House at $263 in the 1990s),[137] the OAPS provides a wealth of primary care medical services to senators, representatives and Supreme Court justices, including physicals, X-rays, physical therapy, and lab work.[138] The Members of Congress do not receive a bill for this care, they do not need to determine which ICD-10 code was used for their medical problem, and they do not need to call their insurance company to consider an appeal. As congressional representatives, it is highly likely that most of them would be challenged to relate to or even understand the medical billing problems of the American patients they represent. While their proclamations, as they run for office, sometimes say that they would like to enact such things like "Medicare for All," none of these representatives ever, *ever*, comment openly about the greatest medical perk possible, the Office of Attending Physician Services.

It is like a secret perk, just reserved for our *special ones*, for our elected representatives. This physician service continues as we hear so much political rhetoric about the desires to "improve medical care" for all

Americans. It is not likely that we can ever count on our representatives in the House or the Senate to "feel the pain" of physicians buried under an avalanche of ICD-10 codes, nor will they experience their patients' struggle to pay their medical bills. It is also highly probable that none of them will feel the challenge of simply trying to find a doctor who does not place bonuses ahead of decent care.

For patients to find one of the few good primary care doctors who is still out there, to find one of those doctors who is increasingly vanishing from the medical landscape of America, would be not just an immense challenge. It would be a worthy and potentially life-saving goal.

Chapter 6

The World

Hippocrates did not just define the standards of medical care for doctors in any one country or any one region in the world. The mandate with his Oath was for the doctors of Greece, Europe, and for all the doctors in the other countries of the world known at that time. More importantly, it became an oath for the doctors caring for patients throughout the world *during the decades and centuries that followed*. Doctors practicing in Africa, in Canada, in the European countries, in Russia and China all have been directed to the same element of obligation for the medical realities before them: the care of people who are suffering from disease, the treatment of patients who are dying, and the relief of symptoms while bringing patients back to a state of good health. Because of this commonality, it was desired for all doctors in all countries to be universally bound by the same Oath...it is a universal statement of morality and obligation for the benefit of the patient. This statement from the ancient writings of Hippocrates is a powerful mandate that, among other essential truths, commands: (*My practice)* ***"will benefit my***

patients according to my greatest ability and judgment, and I will do no harm or injustice to them."

It carries its power to this day for the patients of the world.

What is this element of unity that brings the considerations of Hippocrates to the patients across the globe, and how have the different civilizations responded? As the population of the world has expanded, from the earliest era of human existence through the time of Christ to the teeming civilizations of today, there have been opportunities for unique medical intervention as varied as the populations that seek the best possible care. Dating back in the unwritten history of the medicine men of ancient American Indian tribes to the plains of the Sahara Desert, from a tiny village in Siberia to the former Aztec colonial towns in the Gulf of Mexico, the same need has been replicated as doctors have struggled to understand the best ways to treat the mystical complexities of their patients' diseases.

In the days gone by, the earlier time of Hippocrates and ancient Greece, where something so fundamental as human internal anatomy was virtually unknown, advancements moved slowly through the knowledge that finally became supplied by early autopsies. As time passed, the visual images emerged through the lenses of the microscope that could eventually see the previously-invisible tiny bacterial creatures, advancing further to our intensely detailed electron microscopic pictures of Corona and similar viruses, even now beginning to provide remarkable imaging of such things as brain circuitry as the effects of drugs on the body and the diseases that ravage human cells became better understood. All of this, developing with the emerging understanding of anatomy and physiology, provided the physicians who had launched their careers under the moral guidance of the Hippocratic Oath with the knowledge needed to save lives.

And yet, with the vast variability of the human response to disease, the complex immunologic reactions to pathogens, and the psychological effects in the beleaguered patient with mental disorders, as well as the stress or depression that accompanies disease processes, we continue to study ever more aggressively the most complex and unique elements for all the humans who suffer from disease. Through all this, it is a powerful reality that the doctor, no matter how excellent his or her training, no matter how high the intelligence or how great the experience, never learns it all—he or she simply learns to "practice" *as well as possible* as the knowledge base continues to expand. The physician speaks the Hippocratic Oath upon graduation from medical school and, after more years of specialty training, begins the practice of medicine as the mandates from this oath remain in the background throughout the career. And this presence hopefully continues throughout the doctor's entire professional activity, in every country of the world, leaving each physician having the uncertainty of the cure and the hoped-for benefit of the treatment with the knowledge that he or she fulfilled the mandates of the Hippocratic Oath.

In the practices in all of the countries and in all of the cultures, while the mandates of Hippocrates have remained fundamentally and essentially constant, there have been many different pathways for the doctors seeking of the same goal: the bringing of a cure or the medical benefit to the suffering patient. These variables, superimposed upon the constants of science, give some guidance to what physicians should do to be effective in their care, what patients must do to help the doctor be successful, and what countries must do to allow the best possible care for the citizens struggling with disease.

A look at the different countries and the different medical systems can bring a better understanding of the challenges that face all of us and the elements of commonality that unite us all. First, is there a country where sick patients migrate and seek to enter when they are sick or cannot be cured? Where do sick people go when they need treatment? How much do family members or friends play a role if no physician is available? Next, is there a primary care physician in the town or city *or anywhere* available to see that patient, to respond to the medical symptoms, does that doctor have the background of training and the motivation to effect a cure or at least to provide a significant improvement in the suffering? Looking at the United States, can the care be afforded as we wonder how can it be that every other country in the world delivers healthcare to their population for half the price? And finally, looking at the myriad of medical systems around the world, the remaining question (that can be only partially answered) is in what countries have doctors done it right and have brought their citizens the best possible health, and in what countries do the patients themselves follow fundamental guidelines for their good health that can minimize the *need* for a physician? These questions have been studied and studied again, and yet there continues to be almost as many questions as there are answers.

By looking at the essential question, where has it been done right and what country has the healthiest population, we can start to see trends. Then we can see, in the more successful medical systems of other countries, another question, how can it be done better in our own country? Some elements behind this examination are obvious: there should be more doctors available who can provide care, there must be patients who follow basic health guidelines, and there must be adequate economic standing in the country for the provision of studies and medication to benefit the patient. Although there are many variations in the countries of the world, and within each country, some essential patterns are clear.

****

CHINA AND THE ORIENT

A look into Asia and Eastern medicine reveals a complex history of medical care and various therapies for the entire spectrum of human disease, covering a time span of more than 3,000 years. China has one of the longest recorded histories of medicine records of any existing civilization. The methods and theories of Traditional Chinese Medicine (called "TCM") have developed and repeatedly changed during this time, as Western medical theory and practice came to China in the nineteenth and twentieth centuries, notably through the efforts of missionaries and the Rockefeller Foundation, which together founded the Peking Union Medical College.

Medical care delivered in China historically has depended to a large extent on whether a patient lives in the country or a city. Throughout so much of Chinese history, TCM has been the foundation for healthcare throughout the rural areas of the country. In the second half of the 20th century, after the Communist Party took control of the country's healthcare system, a basic effort was made through state-sponsored systems to send an increasing number of "barefoot doctors"[139] (often farmers, folk healers, rural healthcare providers, and secondary school graduates) into rural communities where city doctors would not offer services.[140] When they were not working in the areas of medical hygiene, family planning instructions, or treating common illnesses, they were often barefoot and working in the rice paddies that covers so much of the land. These individuals largely relied on TCM for much of their treatment. Their traditional medicine depended on herbal treatments, acupuncture, acupressure, moxibustion (burning of herbs over acupuncture points), "cupping" (local suction of skin), qigong (coordinated movement, breathing, and awareness), tui na (massage), and other culturally unique practices. Such approaches were believed to be most effective in treating minor and chronic diseases, in part because of milder side effects. Traditional treatments may also be used for more serious conditions as well, particularly for such acute abdominal conditions as appendicitis, pancreatitis, and gallstones; sometimes traditional treatments are used in combination with Western treatments.

By 1966-1976, during the time of the Chinese Cultural Revolution, Mao Zedong worked to achieve a goal that, for every 1000 Chinese people in the country, one or sometimes two barefoot doctors would be trained. This policy had the advantage of the fact that, these "barefoot" individuals were already working in rural areas, and no additional training was needed; also, their healthcare work was being supplemented by urban doctors who were occasionally sent to the countryside. However, it is notable that these transplanted urban doctors were greatly dissatisfied with their forced displacement and generally considered it to be punishment. The physicians remaining in the cities became government employees as the Chinese government took over complete control of their clinics.[141]

As the displaced doctors merged care with the rural barefoot "doctors," women increasingly entered the profession, allowing the examination and treatment of patients for gynecological conditions, reducing the silent suffering of so many female patients who were reluctant to undergo examinations from male barefoot or displaced urban doctors.[142] As a result, women's health became substantially improved. And so, from all of this, the combination of barefoot doctors (working at medical care when they were not farming) and the displaced doctors practiced a mixture of Western medicine and TCM across the expanse of the China countryside. Funding was reduced for the barefoot doctors on the basis of their agricultural work and generally they were paid about 50% of what one of the more classically-trained doctor earned.

In the rural countryside, caring for the people who could not travel to the urban centers, there was an increasing pattern of "family doctors" traveling to the homes of sick patients, the cost covered by the government.[143] To provide for these healthcare needs, the population of physicians increased; when, in 2005, it was noted that more than 100 million people living in rural areas still had no timely access to medical care, the government initiated another plan, called a "***five-year plan***" and invested more than $2.4 billion in an effort to rebuild rural medical service systems.[144]

In 1981 China reportedly[145] had 516,000 senior physicians trained in Western medicine and 290,000 senior physicians trained in traditional Chinese medicine.

The goal of China's medical professionals has been to try and synthesize the best elements of traditional and Western approaches. If a patient had a mild illness or needed vaccinations, he or she would see the barefoot doctor; for more serious illnesses, the displaced doctors from the cities would see patients, often in "Township Health Centers with 10-30 beds, one clinic for every 10,000-30,000 patients. The most seriously ill were also seen by (often displaced) urban doctors in the County Hospitals; the doctors seeing patients in these facilities had degrees from 5-year medical schools and each was generally responsible for 200,000-600,000 patients, depending on what the magnitude of chronic doctor shortages existed and how many patients with severe illnesses were seeking care.

However, 1981 was the year the barefoot doctor system was abolished and the "barefoot" term was changed to "village doctors," solidified in 1985 by the Chinese Medical Reformation. This allowed these individuals to begin charging patients as the government played a smaller role in national health care. Regretfully, as epidemics began to sweep the Chinese countryside, yet *another* government-directed "***New Rural Cooperative Medical Scheme***" (RCMS) was initiated, and the program was run like an insurance program, covering as much as 90% of the population.[146] This new system allowed about 800 million rural residents to have basic, tiered medical coverage, while the government covered as much as 80% of medical expenses. The system allowed for widespread primary care to the Chinese countryside, and has been given credit for substantially lowering childhood mortality and improving life expectancy to that approaching that of Western modern societies. These improvements also spread to urban communities, and by 2011, more than 95% of the total population of China (currently 1.393 billion people) had basic health insurance, although there were many variations in the out-of-pocket costs and the quality of the care.

Currently, then, Chinese healthcare is a combination of rural and urban care, public and private medical institutions, low-level and advanced-level trained medical personnel, and increasingly widespread insurance coverage. The people living in urban areas are not provided with free healthcare, and are required to either pay for treatment (in advance of receiving that treatment) or purchase health insurance.[147] Under the latest effort to improve urban healthcare in China, *another* initiative was developed, the "***Healthy China 2020 plan,***" requiring insurance to cover 70% of costs.[148] In major cities, many of the hospitals are currently foreign-run ventures of Western-style medical systems with international staff available in several of the larger cities. Patients living in these cities also have access to three different levels of healthcare: factories and neighborhood "Health Stations," and for more serious diseases, "District Hospitals," and then "Municipal Hospitals" for the most critical health issues.

Again, as the more well-trained physicians in these upper-level facilities are siphoned off by the government into rural communities, the pervasive physician shortage for the urban communities became exacerbated. Furthermore, these more advanced hospitals are expensive, and treatment may cost as much as 10X as much as the care in public (District) hospitals which are also available in all Chinese cities, with lower-level and variable quality. A unique component of the public hospitals, however, is how many of them have a so-called V.I.P. ward (Chinese: 高干病房）where more modern technology is available and services are provided to foreigners with doctors and nurses who speak English.

To this day, however, there remains a substantial shortage of doctors and nurses in China. The quality of the diagnostic capabilities and treatment outcomes was determined to be low among primary healthcare physicians.[149] These challenges have been exacerbated by a remarkable process known as "ticket resale" where "tickets" for gaining advanced outpatient consultations that are routinely sold by hospitals for 200 Yuan are being sold on a black market for as much as 3,000 Yuan.[150] At the same time, businessmen are running for-profit ambulance services, often without adequately trained operators and no medical equipment.[151]

Long before Hippocrates proclaimed his moral mandates for treatment, a wide array of "therapies" were being performed with the intent of helping the suffering patient. Although I had attended autopsies at LA County Medical Center while I was a pre-medical student and had seen many unusual causes of death, the most shocking scene came *after* I became a physician. Having graduated from Geffen School of Medicine at UCLA, I had thought I had at least heard of most diseases and treatments of human conditions. I had pledged the Hippocratic Oath, I had graduated, and the next day I had started my year of internship, back in the same vast LA County Medical Center where I had watched autopsies, five years before. After completing a month of remarkable intensity on the 13th floor Jail Ward,[152] I rotated through Pediatrics, and in the middle of a busy clinic day, the senior Pediatric resident walked up to me and asked if I would like to see something I would "probably never see again."

"Of course!" I replied as she led me to another part of the pediatric pavilion.

"This is the pediatric morgue, so to speak," she said with uncharacteristic seriousness as we passed through the door leading into a sealed-off area of the Pediatric Pavilion. It was a cold and somewhat darkened area with three steel tables of varying lengths spanning the center of the room. Lying on the smallest table was the body of an expired Asian boy, about four years of age, with skin that was remarkably dark blue. We stood quietly at the side of the body for a few moments while I tried to think of any question that might sound reasonably intelligent.

"Why is his body so blue?" I finally asked at about the same moment I began to notice several streaks of areas of what looked like burns over parts of his chests.

"Probably strep," she answered, "and he had a high fever before he died. The blue is the consequence of the infection that started the whole thing, something you may remember from medical school, HSP?"

"Henoch-Schönlein purpura?" I responded as she nodded. "From bleeding under the skin?"

"Correct, inflamed and leaking blood vessels, high fever from the strep, probably started as a minor upper respiratory infection. Notice anything else?" she asked.

"Those streaks?" I pointed at his chest. "What are the streaks?"

"Those are the result of *coining*," she said softly, shining her pen light on a group of the streaks, extending down to the boy's abdomen. "The parents are Vietnamese...."

"They did something with coins on the skin?"

"Heated oil on the skin, with the edge of coins scraped across the oil-covered skin, to burn out the fever," she answered. "An ancient Vietnamese folk remedy called 'çao gio,'[153] still used by many American-Vietnamese to try and treat fevers and disease, especially when they can't get a doctor, or as in this case, if they decide to not call a doctor. Also, the coining is practiced by the Chinese, called 'gua sha' and other South Eastern Asian countries such as Indonesia where they call it 'kerikan.' The important thing is that it is not child abuse, it is the cultural efforts of parents to rid the child of fever."

She glanced up at me, and said softly, "It is a cultural thing, a desperate effort to save the child from his disease. This is from parents with an absence of medical knowledge and deciding to proceed with the application of traditional treatment."

The family treatment for this child was clear. Their child had a fever and, after the indoctrinated parent dismisses "modern Western healthcare," as potentially merciless and unfeeling, and not available outside an emergency room, a coining treatment is initiated with high hopes. In India, this may be combined with prolonged consultations and other efforts that include various traditional treatment techniques and herbal additions. After lubricating the skin of the suffering patient with heated oil, often camphor, a hard object such as a coin or piece of jade is forcefully rubbed back and forth until redness ("ecchymosis" from bleeding under the skin) begins to occur. It is believed that the more ecchymosis created, the more releasing of trapped "heatiness" occurs, helping lower the fever. This, of course, involves pain, and depending on how much lubricant is placed, the consequence may even involve burns or camphor toxicity. However, if the fever then dissipates, the treatment is believed to have worked and the family will pass on the success of this coining treatment to the next generation in future years. And so, it carries on from family to family over a time span of many centuries. Importantly, it is often the parent who has the culturally-appropriate "bedside manner" and who may be acutely moralistic in the best traditions of Hippocrates.

And so, with coining, I was introduced to one small part of Asian medical culture. While fundamental comparisons between Western medicine and "Traditional" (or Asian) medicine highlight the often incompatible differences between the two spheres of patient treatment, there are actually some similarities. The Western medical concept of "First, Do No Harm" (*primum non nocere*) would seem to be a premier Western moral theory guiding behavior and therapy, a centerpiece for the promise of Hippocrates. However, virtually everything done with Western medical care actually violates the "do-no-harm" concept. When a Western MD does something as fundamental as injecting an influenza or Covid vaccine into a patient, the potential of infection at the injection site (rare but not impossible) is mitigated by a sterilizing swipe across the overlying skin. Other risks from vaccination such as the rare paralytic Guillain-Barré syndrome (GBS) risk are also disregarded. This risk (about one or two additional GBS cases per million people vaccinated against the flu) contrasts against more than 34,000 deaths from the flu in the United States last year.[154] First, the doctor wants to do some good (prevent influenza and prevent death) while trying to do no harm (by creating potential infection or paralysis); these are two paired entities, where in almost every case of inoculation, the magnitude of benefit is prominently favorable compared to the potential harm from the vaccination. In recent times, this contrasting of benefit and risk of vaccination has been the centerpiece of medical conferences, government mandates, and endless personal conversations.

Looking at a more extreme example of risk and benefit, the large potential of injury from chemotherapy or radiation treatment of advancing cancer, contrasts with something much worse, a potential *death* from the cancer. A doctor, whether in China or in Western countries, looking at each trade-off for each element of therapy, makes the decision to treat *in spite of the potential for harm*. In the litigious world of Western medicine, expanding elements of pretreatment advisories are given a nod that expands to a written acknowledgement with more toxic therapies, theoretically protecting the doctor from a lawsuit.

In contrast, with Traditional Chinese Medicine, the person treating a patient will balance risks based on the *historical beliefs of benefit* passed on through hundreds of generations over a time span of thousands of years. Foremost in the minds of everyone in China is also to initiate a cure in spite of the risk of creating harm, again, a modification of the idealistic element of do-no-harm. Also, this "treating" person, especially in rural areas, is often a family member rather than a physician, using methods handed down by parents, grandparents, and on up the cultural chain.

Today Chinese traditional medicine therefore continues alongside Western medicine and traditional physicians (who also receive some Western medical training). Various traditional preventative and self-healing techniques such as qigong, which combines gentle exercise and meditation, are widely practiced as an adjunct to professional health care. The parents or other relatives living in cities often will fall back on home care, rather than the hospital that is more available in larger cities, using the historical methodology to return the individual to good health. In this setting, the relatives providing established treatment strongly believe in such treatment, and this belief is transmitted to the patient in the same manner as the white-coated bedside presence a prestigious Western physician might provide. This bedside manner reassurance by the provider, as treatment is initiated, actually benefits the patient, remarkably whether the treatment has been established by controlled double-blind scientific trials or by 3,500 years of Chinese precedent. This benefit (from the provider's attitude rather than necessarily by the treatment) is known as the placebo effect and its benefit is relied upon by all providers in the United States as well as in Indonesia, China, Vietnam and other Asian countries. At the same time, this placebo effect is regularly seen in Western scientific trials, and it is recognized that the placebo may actually provide significant benefit to a suffering patient. The intentions of these family members is to help the ill patient come close to the moral proscriptions of the Hippocratic Oath.

This placebo effect, long considered to be a fake benefit in Western medicine, is now being reexamined as an actually important benefit, since the mind of the patient receiving the placebo appears to be able to become a "healing" tool when given the opportunity. Professor Ted Kaptchuk probably said it best from his studies that focused on this phenomenon from the Harvard-affiliated Beth Israel Deaconess Medical Center:

“The placebo effect is more than positive thinking — believing a treatment or procedure will work. It's about creating a stronger connection between the brain and body and how they work together.” And so, doctors in the world of Asian medicine will use these techniques established by this culture. Coining is one of those treatments, easily dismissed by Western licensed physicians as not being evidence-based and therefore having no merit. However, the benefits, as seen by the treating individual, have been described by the ancestors and so scientific proof is not felt to be needed. How harmful can coining be, the family member in Vietnam might ask, as the child lies in bed with a high fever and the bottle of camphor or the containers filled with herbals and other substances are retrieved from the shelf?

The Chinese treatment philosophy is vastly more complicated than any *primum non nocere* concept. The family instructions, or the Traditional treating doctor, will recall such things inherent with the culture as the balance of forces with the known illness from “blocked energy channels.” These channels (the “qi”), together with the balance of energy (the “yin” and the “yang”), and finally the Five Elements, the "Wu Xing"—jin (metal), mu (wood), shui (water), huo (fire), and tu (earth) are believed to act as the foundation of everything in the universe.[155] When it is known that these five characters can generate or destroy each other, if they are applied for a patient's benefit, such trivial side effects as doing some *slight* harm from coining, or from the toxicities of an herbal substance, are of little regard and the method of ridding a patient of fever is still widely practiced among Asians.

Coining is, of course, only a small aspect of traditional Asian medicine, and many in China are not aware of this method of treating fever. In the meantime, the vast spectrum of acupuncture, massage, cupping therapy, herbal medicine, and dietary therapy is dismissed by many with a Western medicine background as "pseudoscience" practices that violate the foundation of scientific trials. Such trials require proof in the West, determined by "double-blinded experiments" where neither the patient nor the doctor knows if a particular treatment is the actual medical substance or a bland placebo. The results of the two groups are then compared and statistical differences are sought. This methodology was, of course, extensively employed in the Covid-19 vaccination trials by numerous pharmacological companies but is difficult with Asian medicine since a true (unaware) placebo group cannot exist when most of these TCM activities are performed.

In contrast, the basic principle of the Chinese and Asian treatments relates to concepts that are not proven by any such rigorous testing experiments. As I have noted, this proof is not needing to confirm the effectiveness of any such treatment since the procedures have already been proven, in the Oriental way of thinking, by the tests of time and tradition. Doctors practicing the TCM treatment, without such blinded testing and with disregard to any "placebo label," are believed to involve interaction with the patient's "circulating channels of branched meridians that connect to body organs and functions." This follows texts such as those found, like a medical bible, in the ancient Chinese text, *Huangdi Neijing*,[156] which emphasize dynamic processes similar to European humoral theory, where health is determined by the balance of those same four humours that are believed to compose the human body: blood, yellow bile, black bile, and phlegm.[157] These writings are considered to be the fundamental source of Chinese medicine, and the two texts comprising this work provide a fascinating question-and-answer format with medical questions being asked of the mythical "Yellow Emperor" and several of his legendary ministers.[158]

And so, in China where this vast array of medical history and direction has been firmly established, what is the family supposed to do for a suffering child or other relative? Can the loving family resolve the illness with the application of TCM? Can doctors be trusted and do doctors in training in China speak the Hippocratic Oath? Do they believe in the moralistic concepts of the oath? A review[159] of the subject several years ago indicated that medical students at more than 120 Chinese medical institutions do take an oath of sorts, but it is considerably different from that of Hippocrates; the oath is spoken during the opening ceremonies by medical student freshmen who are believed to have "absorbed the spirit of the Hippocratic Oath and the Declaration of Geneva." Their oath reads as follows:

The moment I step into this hallowed medical institution, I pledge solemnly-

§ I will volunteer myself to medicine with love for my motherland and loyalty to the people.

§ I will scrupulously abide by medical ethics, respect my teachers and discipline myself.

§ I will strive diligently for the perfection of technology and for all-round development of myself.

§ I'm determined to strive diligently to eliminate human suffering, enhance human health conditions and uphold the chasteness and honor of medicine.

§ I will heal the wounded and rescue the dying, regardless of the hardships.

§ I will always be in earnest pursuit of better achievement. I will work all my life for the development of the nation's medical enterprise as well as humankind's physical and mental health.

Related to this oath is a sad note regarding the fate of Chinese Doctor Li Wenliang in early 2020 after contracting Covid-19 in Wuhan, China, and after having tried to send messages to fellow physicians warning of the lethal nature of the virus. He was quickly ordered by police to "Stop making false statements," and he was then investigated by the communist government for "spreading rumors." Prevented from further warnings, Dr. Wenliang became ill himself from the disease, and he then rapidly deteriorated and died without being able to finalize his efforts to warn the other doctors and the world. Perhaps the first statement in the Chinese medical oath, saying *"...with love for my motherland and loyalty to the people"* allows such control...from a "motherland" that is so tightly regulated by the Chinese Communist Party.

Throughout China, therefore, there are no "private doctors" available for scheduling care for most of the population, and contact for medical care is not initiated by telephone for any reason. No appointments to see a doctor are made—people may see "public" doctors only if they enter the more expensive Western clinic facility. If a patient has a symptom of some infection or other disease, that individual must come to the clinic-like setting where choices are made by the patient between different levels of care; a so-called Grade A hospital with a senior physician may cost $15.00-$20.00, compared to $2.00-$3.00 at the lowest ranked (Grade C) hospital.[160] The Chinese patient is often inclined to see a lower ranked (and less expensive) doctor if the problem is not severe, while a visit to a senior physician in a Grade A hospital would be initiated if a condition seemed to be more severe or life threatening. The waiting time to see a doctor is variable, but an hour wait or sometimes much more, is not unusual.[161]

Care in the hospital setting is always paid for in advance.[162] If care has been given, and further procedures, like the cleaning of ear canals for example, are recommended, it is mandatory that payment for the advanced treatment be provided *before* the treatment will be initiated. If surgery is necessary, an additional payment for the surgery is required before the surgery will be started; without this advance payment, no surgery is allowed. If an "annual" physical exam is desired, a patient will have to pay for it in advance unless his or her place of employment covers the cost. Again, appointments for an annual exam cannot be made and a patient must first enter the hospital, announce a request for a comprehensive exam, pay for the exam (unless covered by an employing company), wait for an available doctor, and then finally receive the exam. Medications are provided within the hospital setting...if a prescription is provided by a treating doctor, the needed drugs are obtained inside that same hospital facility (again, paid for in advance). A follow-up examination is never scheduled, the facility tells you when to return; it is up to the patient to show up at that time; there are no appointments, no reminders, and no preliminary expectations of a visit. In the meantime, if there is an emergency where travel to the clinic would be a problem, the number 120 is called, similar to the 911 call in the United States, and an ambulance may be sent.

Interestingly, in China, there is no hospital care for "homeless" patients or anybody else who is unable to pay in advance...there is no "Medicaid" system for the indigent and, by following this policy, it has been established that there is no "homeless problem" in China.... A large number of Chinese citizens without homes are children, and currently there are about 1 million homeless children, about half of them runaways from abusive or impoverished households.[163] Also, it is important to recognize that Chinese patients rely, far more than in Western countries, on family members for the provision of care. Often the traditional herbs that resolve medical problems are provided by family members in the home setting; if they don't work, the patients with no financial holdings can't walk into their medical facility and demand evaluation or treatment without paying. In this circumstance, a family member with financial reserves will hopefully be found since the State will not pay for the indigent patient without money...care will not be scheduled or delivered. Furthermore, if hospitalization is required for those who *are* able to pay, the family usually brings in food for the patient since the hospital food is generally considered to be tasteless and inferior. If a patient has to remain in the hospital, he or she expects and hopes to receive additional family services, like family members sleeping with the patient, visiting any time of the day or night, turning of the patient, and even some bathing treatments or cleaning activity. Nurses in the hospital are primarily used to provide medications and injections, not to do so much personal care activities as is customary in Western hospitals.

If a Chinese patient experiences an adverse medical condition, and home care cannot be initiated, which hospital facility should he or she visit for care, a Chinese hospital (with Chinese doctors) or a Western hospital (with Western doctors)? Often, the patient will visit one system (more frequently the Western system which may outnumber the Chinese system by a 5:1 ratio). And, if the patient does not improve, he or she will then often go to the *other* system...almost like using the alternate system to obtain a second opinion, with treatment thereafter. There is also, regularly, a choice between Western or Chinese medications; the Western medication is generally much more expensive compared with the Chinese.

If patient in China or Vietnam is being seen by a senior family member, or by a prestigious TCM care doctor in a Chinese clinic, and he or she is then advised about "circulating channels of branch meridians" and the benefits of coining, or perhaps herbal medicine, or cupping, or acupuncture, is it possible that the patient would experience alterations in brain function that can minimize suffering? This might occur by the liberation of "feel-good" neurotransmitters, like dopamine or endorphins, or it may involve changes in mood or emotional reactions that may easily have a therapeutic benefit. As Dr. Kaptchuk said, "The placebo effect is a way for your brain to tell the body what it needs to feel better."[164] Perhaps this underlying mechanism accounts for the success of TCM that might otherwise be dismissed. And, if this positive result did occur, would it not be worthwhile to believe that this is a good thing?

The two branches of healthcare in China persist, as Western procedures and treatments were introduced so many years ago, and it is a matter of debate and discussion as to which branch is predominant for today's Chinese citizen. However, well-informed observers believe that the dominant form of medicine in China today is Western.[165]

RUSSIA

In Russia, medical care is considerably different from that experienced in China or Indonesia. It was declared in the Constitution of the Federation, back in 1996 that all Russian citizens would have the right to "free" healthcare. However, the population has suffered from three elements that challenge the delivery of decent care: a marked shortage of trained physicians, a decline in the allotment of rubles for healthcare, and a relative high level of mortality in the working population, especially in males.[166] During the past couple of years, the number of doctors available to care for the Russian population declined to less than 50 per 10,000 urban citizens (but only 12 per 10,000 citizens in rural populations), a sharp contrast to the United States where nearly 300 physicians are available for the same number of people.[167] [168] During the past ten years, the financial crises in Russia, from the declining value of oil, embargoes by other countries (such as the United States), and inflation, especially in 2014, there has been a plummeting of government money available for healthcare, now only 6.5% of the Gross Domestic Product (GDP), compared with nearly 20% of the

GDP in the United States.[169] Also challenging for the Russians is the mandatory medical insurance deductions from salaries, money taken as a tax from workers to fund nearly half of the medical expenditures. While there is a widespread suspicion that workplace morbidity is high, numbers are difficult to track because only fatalities are reported.

And, with that depressing data for Russian healthcare, how is a citizen supposed to see a doctor in Russia when a medical crisis develops? Considering the prominent uncertainty of finding a doctor, some citizens (about 5%) opt for allowable "private" health insurance. The cost for care under this insurance is very low, $25-$50 for a consultation with a private GP or specialist and between $150-$700 for private treatment, while the cost for an overnight stay in a "private" hospital is between $50 and $100.[170] Personal reports from citizens of Russia indicate the usual pattern of care, when illness occurs, is the patient "goes to the clinic" where care may be obtained, and then the waiting time begins. The waiting time at a clinic is variable depending on the number of patients needing help and the severity of each patient's condition but sometimes stretches into hours. Many patients will stockpile a large amount of medications at home as a personal supply for self-administration as needed, lessening the need for clinic visits. Overnight and prolonged stays in some hospitals can be challenging, and food delivery to inpatients may be required from relatives, similar to the experience noted in China. If an emergency exists, a patient can dial 112 (the Russian equivalent of 911 in the United States), and an ambulance, possibly even with a doctor, can deliver an insured patient to a private hospital. Since emergency calls are answered by Russian-speaking operators, fluency in the Russian language is helpful to allow communications; this can create great difficulties for visitors who do not speak the language.

The doctors I spoke with during a western Russian city visit seemed well-trained, professional, and knowledgeable. Much of their working environment in a small hospital, however, was remarkably archaic; for example the emergency room had one defibrillator and was located at the end of a long and steep staircase. The operating room equipment used glass containers that harkened back to an earlier time. The educational requirement for a Russian to obtain a MD degree is about 6 years; the ethical mandates and morality of the Russian doctor is emphasized by a required oath at graduation from medical training that was established in 1992, the verbiage of which bears a remarkable similarity to the Hippocratic Oath. This replaced the previously approved 1971 oath (that had been called "The Oath of the Soviet Physicians," binding physicians to the principles of "communist morality," an entirely different standard). The newly created oath, "The Promise of Russian Physicians" emphasized the duty of the physician to the individual patient rather than to the Soviet state, and seemed to better reflect the ideals of the Hippocratic Oath for the suffering Russian patient.

The current oath reads:

I SOLEMNLY PROMISE:

To regard him who has taught me the art of doctoring as equal to my parents and to help him in his affairs and if he is in need;

To impart any precepts, oral instruction, and all other learning to my pupils who are bound by the obligation of medical law but to no one else;

I will conduct my life and my art purely and chastely, being charitable and not causing people harm;

I will never deny medical assistance to anyone and will render it with equal diligence and patience to a patient of any means, nationality, religion, and conviction;

No matter what house I may enter, I will go there for the benefit of the patient, remaining free of all intentional injustice and mischief, especially sexual relations;

To prescribe dietetic measures and medical treatment for the patient's benefit according to my abilities and judgment, refraining from causing them any harm or injustice;

I will never use my knowledge and skill to the detriment of anyone's health, even my enemy's;

I will never give anyone a fatal drug if asked nor show ways to carry out such intentions;

Whatever I may see and hear during treatment or outside of treatment concerning a person's life, which should not be divulged, I will keep to myself, regarding such matters as secret;

I promise to continue my study of the art of doctoring and do everything in my power to promote its advancement, reporting all my discoveries to the scientific world;

I promise not to engage in the manufacture or sale of secret remedies;

I promise to be just to my fellow doctors and not to insult their persons; however, if it is required for the benefit of a patient, I will speak the truth openly and impartially;

In important cases I promise to seek the advice of doctors who are more versed and experienced than I; when I myself am summoned for consultation, I will acknowledge their merit and efforts according to my conscience.

If I fulfill this Oath without violating it, let me be given happiness in my life and art. If I transgress it and give a false Oath, let the opposite be my lot.

If you happen to be in Moscow, and have a computer handy, it is not difficult to access doctors in medical centers scattered around the city. For example, the Yauza Medical Center referral system is available online, and if you already know your diagnosis, you can plug it in (about 75 diagnoses are available) and/or if you want a procedure, the desired procedure can be found in the hundreds available. It is therefore possible to access any number of primary care or specialty doctors through the internet although the availability, the cost, and the potential time delays are not defined.[171] Interestingly, an alphabetical list of prominent and notable medical doctors in Russia is also available in Wikipedia,[172] including one unique surgeon who actually performed an appendectomy on himself during an Antarctic expedition and another doctor who was the oldest practicing physician in history, retiring at the age of 103. The practical value of this information for a suffering patient trying to find a doctor is, of course, highly limited.

UNITED KINGDOM

Even after the expansion of Great Britain's empire into the colonial vastness of North America, medical care continued in England as it had through the Dark Ages hundreds of years before. Throughout the 18th century, the people within the United Kingdom suffered almost as much from the *spread* of disease as they did from the *treatments* of disease that were available from the physicians of that time.[173] The concept of bacteria (and associated need for hygiene and cleanliness) was, of course, unknown. One of the greatest fears was malaria, spread by the mosquitos in the marshlands of England, and the belief then was that the disease was spread from a poisonous gas (called "miasma") that regularly wafted up into the atmosphere from sewers and so-called cesspits. During those years, the residents and visitors described the 'marsh fevers' of those areas, variously calling them 'agues', 'tertian fevers', 'quartan fevers' or 'intermittent fevers', consistently attributing them to the noxious poisonous gas rather than to the anopheles mosquito loaded with the malaria parasite. The parasitic nature of malaria was not discovered until 1880, as the previously noted four humours described in blood were, as before, believed to rule the body.

The physicians, who were certainly familiar with Hippocrates, tried to cure people using such things as fox lungs (for asthma) as well as a potpourri of spider's webs, live worms, swallows' nests, and even the skulls of executed criminals ground up into various potions for everything else. The miracle critter, blood-sucking leeches, was used regularly to reduce blood pressure, and to cure most other disease that afflicted the population. The leeches were even bred for the blood-letting purpose, with as many as 6 million being used annually, the amount of blood being removed as much as 80% of the patient's blood[174] if the disease was felt to be serious and life was at risk. It was believed that the leeches, by removing the blood, would remove the toxins that caused disease. Leeches were slow, however, and by venous needles the blood-letting could be, and often was, accelerated. This more rapid blood-removal concept was even carried to the American colonies where, in 1799, a deathly-ill George Washington was bled by his physicians on four occasions during the same day (without leeches), removing 40% of his total blood[175] over 12 hours, followed by (and possibly causing) the retired President's death shortly thereafter.[176]

The doctors of Great Britain also struggled with herbs to resolve medical problems. Although most were useless and without known medical benefit, as previously noted, the Foxglove plant (containing Digoxin) was used following its discovery in 1775, and the herb wintergreen was found to relieve pain and to reduce inflammation. It was not known for centuries that the wintergreen contained the chemical salicin, a primary ingredient of aspirin (salicylic acid). Women giving herbs to suffering patients unfortunately faced the risk of being labeled as "witches," especially if the herbs worked well, and they would then be occasionally put to death by hanging or drowning. Another opportunity for the suffering patient was always the chance of a "royal touch" where an English king could touch a patient's neck near an inflamed tuberculosis gland and, if the TB went into remission, the king was given credit for a cure. During the previous century, King Charles II touched more than 92,000 suffering patients, over 4,500 annually,[177] and the population cheered as many thereafter seemed to be cured as they moved into remission. The King's Touch even seemed to be more effective than the best physicians of that time in resolving disease.

Throughout Great Britain, the treatment of human afflictions was even more challenging because of the lack of rudimentary knowledge about the human body. The church had continued the prohibition of cutting open a human body after death and so basic knowledge of human anatomy was not available. This persisted for many years even in the first institutes of medical training like the University of Edinburgh Medical School, founded in 1726, or in those institutes that followed like the one in Glasgow in 1744 or St. George's Medical School, which began formal teaching in 1751.[178] The people of England, therefore suffered from their myriad of diseases much in the same manner as the North America colonial population that had begun to evolve during that time. To further understand the circumstances of medical care in Great Britain, it is helpful to examine the mirror of healthcare of her colonies in North America, along with the suffering of the American Indians, to appreciate how little the feedback from those people helped shape the subsequent English practice of medicine.

As medicine in the world progressed with time and the spread of civilization, the beliefs of Hippocrates always remained in the background, defining ethical doctor behavior. It would seem logical that the colonies in the United States would have developed a system of doctors and treatment derived from our country's English heritage...until one thinks of the Revolutionary War. This "War of Independence" is routinely defined as the breakaway of the thirteen original colonies triggered by widespread dissatisfaction of the English crown's policies of taxation as well as the near-absence of colonial representation in England. However, medical care in this country also experienced a breakaway at the time of independence, influenced to some degree by exposure to North American Indian knowledge of American flora for the treatment of numerous conditions suffered by members of the tribes.

As an unfortunate consequence of the English and European colonialists migrating into the New World, the Native Indians of North America became rapidly overcome by the untreatable huge spectrum of new diseases brought into their environment, including such conditions as smallpox, bubonic plague, chickenpox, cholera, the common cold, diphtheria, influenza, malaria, measles, scarlet fever, sexually transmitted diseases, typhoid, typhus, tuberculosis, and pertussis (whooping cough).[179] The arriving carriers of these diseases, while crossing the Atlantic, were often incubating the conditions or were partially asymptomatic, their resistance derived from a long history of society-generated states of partial immunity. However the American Indians, without such immunity, were devastated by these conditions, which were not easily treated or understood by the tribes' Medicine Men. The stark reality of the Indian mortality from British disease is suggested in this 1762 journal entry recording the dialogue from Mary Jemison, a Seneca Indian captive at Ohio's Fort Miami:

Brother, We are very thankful to Sir William Johnson for sending you to enquire into the State of the Indians. We assure you we are Rendered very miserable at Present on Account of a Severe Sickness that has seiz'd almost all our People, many of which have died lately, and many more likely to Die. ... '"The 30th, Set out for the Lower Shawneese Town' and arriv'd 8th of September in the afternoon. I could not have a meeting with the Shawneese untill the 12th, as their People were Sick and Dying every day.[180]

The result of all this morbidity and mortality was that significant amounts of evolving medical knowledge in the colonies never significantly affected or made it in reverse, back to the United Kingdom. While these disease conditions clearly played a role in the American medical evolution, it is notable that, during and prior to the 1700s, healthcare knowledge regularly migrated in the one direction, and one direction only, to the colonies from the other side of the Atlantic. The medical recommendations in America clearly reflected Great Britain's state of medical care, indicating the prevailing consideration that what seemed to work in England should also work in the colonies.

An early example of this may be found in a 1643 book of medical recommendations for the doctors of the colonies. In this book, the governor of the Massachusetts Bay Colony, John Winthrop, was given recommendations by a London physician for treating gunpowder burns, using an ointment that was "Mosse that groweth on an old thackt howse top."[181] This "mosse" was an ingredient that was very common in the British countryside (on rooftops) but not in the colonies, and yet the seemingly-relevant medical recommendations were given by the governor to the residents of Massachusetts, direct from a doctor in London. If Americans determined that moss of any kind, which was difficult to find, actually did not seem to improve gunpowder burns, that knowledge never made it back to England.

Another example from the 1643 book was British medical advice to prevent smallpox by "burning a pot of toads to ash and consuming their remains."[182] The colonial *recommendations* for British and European remedies underscore the depth of how early America medical care followed the British experience before the citizens of an emerging America had the time or experience to adapt and uniquely develop its own unique system of healthcare, and there is little knowledge of any American knowledge then being adapted by the British.

Additionally, physicians like Cotton Tufts, educated at Harvard (founded 1636 in Cambridge), treated his patients with an emphasis on the large number of intellectual authorities involved in his training, each of whom provided a distinct European pattern of medical thought. For example, his recommended treatment of conditions suffered by colonialists such as "fevers and complaints of the stomach and throat," should include, he said, "lime, lemon, sugar in a wine glass," a dialogue suggesting an expanded one-way connection to an emerging North America, through trade routes followed by British ships moving through Caribbean ports.[183] And a Boston physician, Dr. James Lloyd, described many of his cases from his experiences in a London hospital, not any experiences in an American hospital, in the mid-1700s.[184] Finally, one of the founding members of Harvard Medical School, Dr. Benjamin Waterhouse, filled a notebook with a large amount of information he had gathered while attending medical lectures at the University of Edinburgh[185] (in Edinburgh, Scotland, founded in 1582). The British location in which medical doctors learn their profession regularly determined what they teach to medical students in future years, and these medical students continued to practice the English method of treatment, throughout England as well as America.

The payment for medical care in the United Kingdom demonstrated another continued pathway for the English, unaffected by the changes evolving in America. Prior to and after the revolution, the evolving mechanism of payment for medical care in North America differed greatly from the English system. It even differed greatly within itself, depending on where patients lived; in the country payment for care was documented to consist of “a linen handkerchief,” brown sugar, butter, and a bushel of “Ingeon meal,” as well as currency.”[186] Payment for healthcare in the city evolved from workers in a growing professional class (such as chair makers, rope makers, painters, sail makers, bakers and shop keepers), who paid for their medical care in cash. It is not too great a stretch of the imagination to suggest that even “a chicken” might have been considered a useful payment from country residents in England as well as in the developing colonies. None of these payment mechanisms became considered by the British in their continued separate process of financial transactions for medical care.

After the colonial breakaway allowing America to follow its own treatment and payment pathways, Europe continued to move along its own different corridor, and in the United Kingdom, different systems of payment for care developed which greatly influenced how doctors were able to see patients, how physicians were paid for their care, and what considerations of quality medicine could evolve. Four similar but independent systems finally evolved into the mainstay of the United Kingdom medical payment policy, involving the three countries beyond England: Scotland, Ireland, and Wales, and later to some extent, even Canada. This evolved during the decades and centuries after the War of Independence until finally, in 1946, England passed the National Health Service Act, (and a year later Scotland passed the National Health Service Act in Scotland) and all the countries then moving into widespread implementation by 1948.

As the English medical systems became even more firmly established, the individual countries modified their own policies for health care, again resulting in four separate but similar systems. The end result was that the UK government sets the overall budget for England while the other three countries (Wales, Northern Ireland, and Scotland) were allotted "block grants" from England to spend on their health care. This is, then, a National Health Service system (NHS) for the United Kingdom with some local country modifications, and it has been working relatively well since the late 1990s.[187]

In 2012, the English system finally evolved into a "new" organization, known as "NHS England," which is now responsible for day-to-day operations and oversees the multiple organizations that, through primary care doctors, provide healthcare to the citizens. In theory, patients are to have choices about which hospital to go to and which specialist to see, but this has not been fully implemented to date. This system is primarily publicly funded through taxes on the citizens and provides access to private health services providers for a wide range of care. These systems are different in each country in Great Britain, however, they are similar to Canada's social programs for such needs as acute and chronic illness, disability, and conditions inherent to the elderly.[188] Two-thirds of doctors in England remain independent as "private contractors," but like in the United States, they are progressively migrating into networks; there is also a significant increase in salaries, going up by 800% since 2004. In theory there may be some patient choice as to which hospital to visit or which specialist to see, but this is apparently not yet fully operational.[189]

With all of these systems in place for many years now, how well do they work for the citizens who seek care? How closely do the doctors of England and associated countries follow the moral guidance of Hippocrates as they provide care under the controls of the NHS? In the beginning of the lengthy evolution of medical systems, medical scholars in Great Britain were, of course, well aware of the Hippocratic Oath, and in recent years, there has been a trend to return to the original Oath. As we have seen, the Hippocratic Oath is probably one of the best examples of the collaboration between nations, as well as a unity of moral principle between the United States and the United Kingdom. Whereas the oath in Great Britain has been evaluated, modified, brought into use and brought out of use for graduating medical students, it is continuing to withstand most of the considered alterations. Interestingly, at least one British medical school has adopted the twentieth century version of the oath by the American physician and professor at Johns Hopkins University, Louis Lasagna. The number of medical schools in the UK using the actual Hippocratic Oath was only 50% in 1997, but this percent has progressively increased to 70% in 2017.[190]

Personal anecdotes from patients using the UK healthcare system report a generally high level of satisfaction with the NHS in England and Scotland. Finding a doctor in this system can be challenging, however, and patients report difficulty reaching a MD. Also, after a telephone call for help, they report having to wait for prolonged periods before a "call-back" occurs on a "specified day." Once contact with a physician has been made, the progression to appropriate specialty consultants can occur if needed, although further waiting is described, for these specialists are not always available.

In spite of the substantial taxation to maintain the English system, there is a sense of reassurance in most patients in the UK that the NHS is there, and even with its problems, care through this system is generally available if needed. However, many patients are financially able to purchase private medical insurance to gain a more timely response than the NHS pattern of response (although the same physicians often provide care in *both* private and NHS settings). The NHS care has been observed to be "doctors doing what is required" in spite of the pattern of waits and less-than-personal care. In more urgent cases, for example, calling the NHS hotline (NHS-24) will either result in a diagnosis over the telephone or, if there is a clear-cut emergency (such as chest pain), 999 may be called and the operators will send an ambulance.

Since it is reported[191] that weekends and holidays can be particularly challenging in being able to locate a doctor, one of the primary recommendations from Scottish and British patients is "Don't get sick on weekends" when doctor availability is reduced. However, most of the time, the NHS seems to work as a generally reliable system creating some degree of reassurance, even with known delays, and with the uncertainty as to which doctor will become available on any given day (from what is called a "pot luck" patchwork of doctors). There are some significant caveats, however. If a patient in London calls to speak to a doctor, it doesn't work...a receptionist takes the call and passes your call on to a secretary; this requires approximately 15 minutes of waiting "on hold." Then, when you finally do get through, and a request to speak with a physician is made, you are informed that the doctor will call you back. The time delay for this "call-back" is often 2-3 days. Alternatively, if you simply ask for a nurse to take a blood test, that delay can take a week. *Nobody seems to really care that a distressed patient needs to talk with her doctor.* If you decide you need an ambulance, during the long wait to actually speak with a doctor, you have to call *another* number, different from the usual 999 emergency number. The frustrations (and additional disease risks) with this delay may be allayed some by the knowledge that, if you are old enough, you don't have to pay for either drugs or the ambulance, since your ongoing NHS taxation process will "take care of it."

On the other hand, there is a *private* system in Great Britain that functions more like the "Rolls Royce" of medical care with minimal delays and a greater certainty regarding available physicians for acute conditions. Furthermore, while the doctors working under the NHS banner appear to be more fully enveloped by, and preoccupied with, computer management of care, these "private physicians" don't seem to be sidelined by their computers to the same degree. This suggests that the private doctors' bedside manner is significantly better than that found with the NHS system in general. It would seem likely that the private doctors, when working more independently from the government, would feel the Hippocratic calling, *into whatever homes I go, I will enter them for the benefit of the sick*, not re-defined as "except on weekends," or "when I get back to you in a couple of days" as a mandate that speaks louder than the obligations defined by NHS England.

The charges and the costs for medical services in the United Kingdom have evolved from a complex network of financial interactions, mostly covered, as I have noted, the result of substantial taxation upon the citizens. In NHS England, patients are not directly charged for most medical services since they have already paid through the massive and comprehensive taxation system of the country. However, there is a small charge for medicine (about $8.00) unless one is old enough, over the age of 60, when it is "free." If patients decide to obtain insurance to allow for the additional Private Care (for better service, improved choice of specialists, better access to primary care availability and better access to elective procedures), the cost for that insurance is significant, about $1800 per year.[192] However, almost 90% of UK patients do *not* carry such insurance and over 95% of English health care expenditures are from the NHS rather than from private insurance.[193] Although the payment for most of the NHS expenditures comes from general taxes on the citizens, about 20% of NHS payments comes from something they call "national insurance," a polite name for *another* tax on payroll that must be paid by employees and employers.[194] Notably, the private insurance coverage is not comprehensive, and the policies rarely cover medical expenses for maternity care or the costs of mental health care.[195]

Serving the population of the entire United Kingdom, there is a unique and remarkable localized medical presence that has become significant over the past 160 years. Within the city of London, there is a once-unremarkable street running south from Regent's Park with its beautiful Queen Mary's Rose Gardens for about a half mile to a public garden called Cavendish Square. This one-way street was named for the 1767 Lord Mayor of London, Thomas Harley, and since the 1800s, its sidewalks have accumulated a vast collection of medical buildings and expertise for the patients of the United Kingdom. Harley Street originally had about 20 doctors practicing their art in 1860, but the positive environment for an expanding number of patients seeking care created a remarkable growth of doctors willing to supply that care. By 1900, there were about 80 doctors on Harley Street, and by 1914, there were almost 200; their numbers continued to expand ever more rapidly after the years that encompassed World War I and II. When the United Kingdom's National Health Service was established in 1948, there were approximately 1500 doctors on Harley Street, and today this area employs about 3,000 people in a spectacular collection of medical practices, clinics, and hospitals, as well as paramedical practices. The entire area has become a kind of *medical epicenter* for the English citizens, especially in the London area.

Since more than half of the UK's highest earners now live in London[196] as well as the nearby southeast area of England, and since development of luxurious housing and the central proximity to important railway stations are near Harley Street, the area has been a magnet for medical doctors and expanded medical care, albeit overwhelming *private* care. There is also a reputation of attracting services that focus on cosmetic care and fertility services. The result of this "private" differentiation is primarily that a *service* is provided (with less waiting time, a more cordial staff, and a more efficient resolution of problems) contrasting with the NHS and its more robotic and *get-in-line* atmosphere. Many of the doctors practicing on Harley Street also practice within the National Health System and so the *quality* of care is often comparable although the style and efficiency of delivering that care may be greatly different and often more expensive.

CANADA

Any discussion of healthcare in Canada requires an understanding of the Canadian financial morass that evolved as the organized system for payment of medical care developed and evolved.

Medical care in Canada followed similar pathways as those in England and its American neighbor to the south, guided by Hippocratic moral guidelines, while the country continuously struggled to establish a workable method of paying for the care. The process was particularly difficult because of the myriad of differing Canadian humanity, a patchwork of 10 provinces and 3 territories, with patients living in the cities and the remote countryside, spread across the vast territory dispersed from the Atlantic to the Pacific, and each area with individual unique medical concerns and payment challenges. Canadians finally established representation in the House of Commons in 1867 within the Parliament, which closely followed the makeup of the English House of Commons, and the MPs (Members of Parliament) who represent the population much as the members of our own House of Representatives in Washington. Meeting in

Ottawa regularly and struggling with the massive payment-for-care issue, a tentative solution for funding medical services finally was established in 1984 with the passage (unanimously) of the Canadian Healthcare Act (CHA) that profoundly affected how medical care could be delivered to ailing members of the public.

The struggle by the government to deliver and pay for the healthcare of the population had been remarkably tortuous. Trying to change the division of powers between the federal government and the provinces was challenging, requiring an alteration that finally resulted in a constitutional amendment. Over the many years prior to the CHA, the individual provinces had challenged, fought against, and sued the central government's efforts to coalesce them into the single mechanism that the Healthcare Act actually finally achieved…by any measurement, the process of agreeing to a constitutional amendment in Canada was extraordinarily difficult.

Professor Malcolm G. Taylor, at Toronto's York University, probably described the problems best in his book[197] that concisely summarized Canadian healthcare prior to 1984, looking at the seven major decisions leading to the new system, and the results of the final outcome. Efforts had been made to deliver health services by the physicians "privately" for patients, but "administered and funded by the provinces." However, Canadian patients in the different provinces regularly faced disability, accidents, and illnesses that were largely unpredictable, resulting in payments to doctors that were also unpredictable. With these "private" efforts to struggle and pay for medical services by the people who were often sick and unemployed, the physicians working to help them found themselves progressively sinking into such great debt by non-payments that their availability to provide services became increasingly rare. Various efforts to establish provincial social insurance systems regularly failed because of the intense opposition of the provinces to the federal incursions into their healthcare procedures.

Finally, the pressures for a financing system became so great that, under the liberal government led by Joseph Trudeau in 1984, the CHA came into reality and a comprehensive health service system was implemented. "Medicare" is the general term that refers to Canada's publicly funded health care system, and under this system, all Canadian residents ("insured" by the government) have the expectation of reasonable access to medically necessary hospital and physician services without paying out-of-pocket. Insured health services under this act include hospital services, physician services, and surgical-dental services provided to the covered persons. Under the terms of the Canadian Healthcare Act, all "insured persons" are entitled to receive services without copayment. Such services are defined as medically necessary services if provided in the hospital, or by "practitioners" (usually physicians).

The seemingly laudable elements of the CHA were stated in the preamble of the Act, defining the objective of Canadian Health Care policy "to provide continued access to quality health care without financial or other barriers is critical to maintaining and improving the health and well-being of Canadians." To its proponents, this impressive statement sounded noble as they declared: "access to health care should be based on need, not ability to pay...this is the defining national value of Canada."[198] And yet as this "defining national value" that was supposed to allow access to health care, unfortunately turned out greatly different from the ideal.

As noted, the primary objective of the Act was to protect, promote and restore the physical and mental wellbeing of residents of Canada and to facilitate reasonable access to health services without financial or other barriers. To do so, the Act listed a set of criteria and conditions that the ten provinces and three territories must follow in order to receive their federal transfer payments that paid for the care. These items included the regions of *Public Administration, Comprehensiveness, Universality, Portability* (between provinces), and *Accessibility*. The primary objectives of this system were to create a nonprofit administration operated by a public authority, coverage for all insured health services provided by hospitals, physicians or dentists, and the expectation that all of the "insured persons" (almost everybody) would have health services "provided for by the plan on uniform terms and conditions." Remarkably, the definition of actions allowing accessibility and the crucial matter of "payment" were left…undefined.

As the CHA system became implemented, payment to the doctors and to the provinces for healthcare regularly underwent regulatory activity stemming from the Act's provisions that ordered payments to the individual provinces be withheld if (poorly-defined) "overbilling" was detected by the central monitors of such activity. A government bureaucrat then seeking evidence of "overbilling" examined the charges from the doctor and arrived at conclusions that were often greatly at odds from the reality of expenses individual doctors incurred while trying to deliver care.

The official wording of this expanding government control of billing may then be summarized in this challenging bureaucratic edict as follows:[199]

Deduction for extra-billing

20. (1) Where a province fails to comply with the condition set out in section 18, there shall be deducted from the cash contribution to the province for a fiscal year an amount that the Minister, on the basis of information provided in accordance with the regulations, ***determines to have been charged through extra-billing*** *by medical practitioners or dentists in the province in that fiscal year* *or, where information is not provided in accordance with the regulations, an* ***amount that the Minister estimates to have been so charged****.*

Deduction for user charges

20. (2) Where a province fails to comply with the condition set out, there shall be deducted from the cash contribution to the province for a fiscal year an amount that the Minister, on the basis of information provided in accordance with the regulations, ***determines to have been charged in the province (or) an amount that the Minister estimates to have been so charged.***

It is a classic government order of bureaucratic double-speak. The doctors are allowed to charge whatever they want, unless they "overbill." Translation: doctors are allowed to charge only what the government allows and no more. If the "Minister" determines they charge more than the poorly defined government limits, by his or her poorly-defined "estimate," no matter the costs to maintain an office, no matter the costs to pay the doctor's employees, or the costs of malpractice insurance, the government can decide an *infraction* has occurred and then chop the province's payments. At the same time,

Canadian physicians who are in private practice or work for hospitals are *required* to spend additional funds to obtain medical liability insurance, available through the Canadian Medical Protective Association (CMPA). Also, predictably, physician charges quickly climbed and as penalties were levied by the central government, a withholding of medical payments to the provinces quickly followed. A translation of this "withholding" might be the *fining* of the provinces in this strange *"first, we allow, and then we take away"* policy.

The financial consequences to the provinces were profound. Examples of subsequent regulatory activity include financial penalties totaling $246,732,000, withheld from the provinces in the first two years.[200] The bureaucratic burden on physicians to avoid what the government called "extra-billing" or "user charges" quickly became a challenging daily problem as doctors struggled to remain in compliance with the poorly-defined law. Almost predictably, the doctor anger over this "extra-billing" accusation became so contentious that Ontario's physicians broke all precedence of professional behavior and actually went on strike in protest in 1986 (see photo).

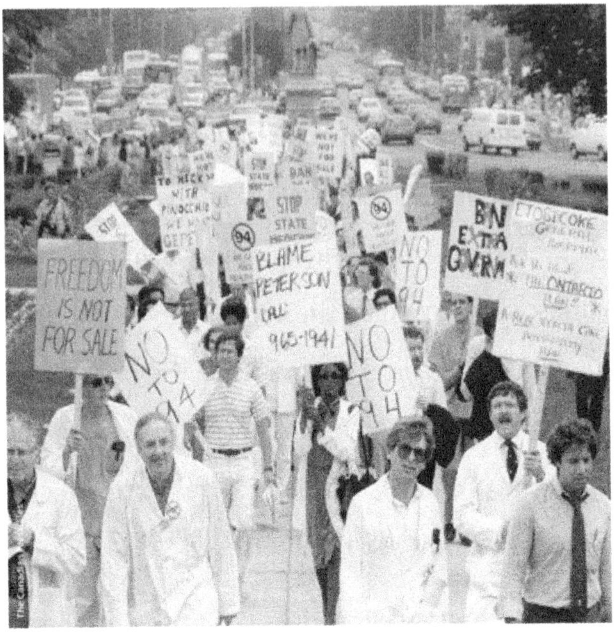

Ontario physicians march on Queen's Park in Toronto, Ont., June 15, 1986, during their strike to protest a government ban on extra-billing. Image courtesy of The Canadian Press/files.

None of this improved much by 1993 when British Columbia finally allowed about 40 doctors to proceed with "extra-billing" in their work for patients. However, the Canadian federal overseers promptly reduced the payments to British Columbia by a whopping $2,025,000.[201] A couple of years later, the Canadian government did the same thing to Alberta's province, reducing their payments by $3,585,000[202] for their expenditures of "user fees" being charged in private clinics. The federal government did the same thing to Nova Scotia (for physicians charging "user fees,") and in a bold move of transient independence, Nova Scotia refused the entire federal transfer payment. To create oversight for the patients (who discovered that doctors were predictably becoming scarce), the Government of Canada published a statement each year outlining how well or poorly each province has complied with the provisions.

For the patients, this helped relieve them of cost (fulfilling the initial concept of the CHA) while, at the same time, challenging them to find an increasingly vanishing doctor in the process. For many patients, the search for a doctor became a medical nightmare. One patient recently reported it took him six years to find a personal physician in the province of Ontario and that, even with a critical red blood cell medical disease, it was nearly impossible to find an available hematologist.[203] While the patients acknowledge that the health care is, for the most part, "free," they point out that this "free" care means a massive shortage of primary care physicians. Furthermore, this increasing shortage of doctors compounds the healthcare problems for the patients when it is combined with some of the longest waiting lists in the world.[204] The problem continues to worsen yearly because of the length of time it takes to train new doctors, leading to progressively more aggressive efforts to recruit an ever-larger number of foreign trained physicians to start new practices in Canada.

This has resulted in the "physician to population" ratio in Canada being almost the worst in the developed world, reaching an embarrassing 26th out of 28.[205] This problem, however, is far worse than embarrassing, since each patient who delays care because of being denied the ability to find a doctor will likely become sicker, *increasing* the demand even more for medical care in a struggling and floundering healthcare system.

And, unfortunately, in the face of this worsening shortage of physicians, the "foreign recruitment effort" has not gone well. Even with the recent Covid-19 epidemic and the increasing fears that patients could not find a doctor, only about 24 new doctor licenses were approved in Ontario in 2020 and none in British Columbia.[206] In a desperate effort to attract new overseas doctors, British Columbia created a "new class" of medical license that allowed foreign doctors to practice under the supervision of a fully licensed Canadian doctor. This has also failed, mainly because the requirements for the new foreign license was poorly communicated to potential applicants.

The net result of these cascades of failures is that Canadians are finding it almost impossible to find a new doctor—currently, there are only 241 physicians serving 100,000 people (compared to the OECD[207] average of roughly 350 physicians per 100,000 patients).[208] However, for patients in the province of Ontario seeking a primary care physician for its 15,000,000 people, only about 100 doctors are available per 100,000 patients.[209]

For doctors in Canada, seeking to take care of patients and follow the moral code defined by the Hippocratic Oath, the overload of patients combined with the government's limitations on what can be charged creates a medical scenario that severely diminishes the doctors' ability to follow the Oath. Also, although the Oath is still administered by many of the 17 medical schools in Canada (14 English, 3 French), the Canadian version of the Oath neglects to mention any reference to a moral obligation for physicians to be honest with their patients[210] and, considering the overload, that omission seems almost intentional. It takes extra time per patient for elements of honesty to be introduced into discussions about medical options...the *recommendation* of any random medical option is much quicker and, when the waiting room is full, anything quicker is important. The moral mandates of the Hippocratic Oath remain strong in the minds of the physicians graduating from Canadian medical schools but the implementation of a single standard of medical care throughout the country became almost impossible.

What is now left brings only three elements of the Hippocratic Oath to be spoken in 80% of the schools' commencement ceremonies:

- respecting confidentiality,
- avoiding harm
- upholding the profession's integrity.

Along with these challenges of declining doctor availability, in this long and convoluted medical history of Canada, the establishment of a comprehensive moral code has undergone a tortuous evolution. Trying to follow international standards for physician morality, most of the existing medical elite in Canada joined together back in 1867 at a conference in Quebec. The purpose of this meeting was to establish a new national medical association and to rid the country of widespread marginal vendors of medicine (quacks), a sincere effort to establish a national standard of doctor ethics. However, one of the physicians of that era, Dr. Charles Tupper, who had been the former Premier of Nova Scotia, made the remarkable comment, *"I do not believe that any elaborate code of medical ethics is required.... The professional man who stands by that golden rule will exhibit in all his dealings, both with his professional brethren and the community at large, the character of the true gentleman, and will require little else, I believe, for his guidance."*[211] He noted that his American-trained Canadian physician colleagues were in the process of modifying the AMA "Code of Ethics" to suit Canadian needs, with the result that Canadian doctors were expected to exemplify "Christian moral character."[212]

Following this initial effort, and between 1868 and 1996, a total of 19 continuously-revised "Codes of Ethics" were formulated. It seems the best medical brains in the country struggled to get it right with regards to morality. The first Code of Ethics (in 1868) was 13 pages long; by 1922, this code had been reduced to 7 pages, and finally by 1996, the code was 4 pages long. To move from 13 pages of morality to 4 pages in 128 years suggests that ethical standards might be adversely affected by extraneous forces and could be significantly declining in quality. A detailed analysis of the evolution of medicine in Canada during these years[213] points out the challenges caused by the fact that, unlike physicians in the Greek society of Hippocrates, there is the inherent conflict between the aura of altruism and the realities of self-interest (financial challenges) that are inherent in any modern medical practice.

Finally, in 2018, the now revised seven-page Canadian Code of Ethics[214] defined the expected moral standards of a physician practicing in the provinces across the country. This is the closest document in Canada to follow the elements of the Hippocratic Oath, and it clearly describes the principle elements of an ethical medical practice. Defining the important qualities of Compassion, Honesty, Humility, Integrity, and Prudence, this code lays out the hallmarks of ethics, while outlining the "Fundamental Commitments of the Medical Profession." And, the final element of the code almost redefines the Hippocratic Oath as the Canadian doctor's professional responsibilities.

As a fundamental shift in society, moving from Greek feudalism (with its levels of social class) to the modern world of capitalism with Western democracy exemplified by the massive payment schemes from insurance companies and governments, the purity that defined the essence of the Hippocratic Oath became altered. And, for the Canadians, the diminishment of the Hippocratic Oath, now replaced by the Code of Ethics, together with the problems associated with the government determining what can and cannot be charged for medical care, has evolved into an ever-worsening doctor shortage and increased patient suffering.

Has the time arrived for another re-evaluation of the physician ethics for the patients of Canada, perhaps a model that will eliminate these problems of doctor shortages that continuously expand across the country? Since the Canadian formulators of ethics appeared inclined in 1868 to follow the revising labors of the United States led by the American Medical Association's Code of Ethics, perhaps revisions may emerge from so many people who are seeking better medical availability and care.

We have seen from the closer examinations of other countries in the world, there is a wide spectrum of policies that govern the medical care patients may receive. From the experiences of the United States, China, Russia, the United Kingdom, and Canada, patterns have emerged over the past couple of centuries suggesting the evolution of an underlying constant that has evolved since the time of Hippocrates. Further studies of the European states, of medical care in Australia, in New Zealand, Japan and Singapore show similar patterns indicating this "constant" for medical care throughout the civilized world, achieving a fundamental need and philosophy. It seems like the issue of a country trying to create decent medical care for its citizens faces three conflicting elements: how to train enough physicians, how to pay for care delivered to the largest possible number of patients, and how to allow those patients (perhaps 10%) who are financially secure and want *better* (more efficient or timely) care than the country's government can supply, while still being taxed for the government version of care. China and Southeast Asia have a fourth variability resulting from their remarkable thousands of year's history of less-expensive "Traditional" care that is imbedded in their healthcare delivery system.

It is, of course, a reality that patients live highly variable lives with many degrees of health and life expectancies. And, these patients have universal experiences and hopes for being able to access care without crushing expenses. Governments have established commendable goals of delivering what is often termed as "free" care to a large portion of their population, the costs buried in different taxation systems that allot payments for variable amounts of services as citizens endure often-crushing or increasing tax burdens. In the effort to accommodate the varying expectations of a population having such a wide spectrum of health needs, with so many variables in patients' financial statuses and such a wide range of ages and social burdens, patterns or mandates have emerged in virtually all the countries of the world:

1. Government policy will ensure medical care will be available to all citizens regardless of their ability to pay, and repeatedly, this care will be characterized as "free."
2. Since the available resources to provide medical care to the *entire* population is limited, there will be crowding experiences for people who possess little or no money and who access this "free" care, and there will be increased costs (taxation) experienced by those with higher financial capabilities.
3. Emergency care will always be available regardless of the ability to pay. It follows, of course, that if *ongoing medical care* is not adequately being provided, the emergency care will be required more often than would otherwise be needed.
4. Patients with increased resources will pay more, often much more, in the form of increased taxes on their earnings and holdings, and increased costs for the premiums on insurance; this may then allow

for improved doctor availability, reduced waiting times, and improved services for those patients.

5. The government regulation of charges for medical care will be used to constrain patients' money paid for examinations and procedures, using criteria that is at the same time all-encompassing and often illogical (think ICD-10), while trending toward becoming endlessly expansive.
6. There will be, as a result of the above, increasing physician shortages especially in primary care, and it is virtually certain that delivered care will be significantly unequal for the population.

The governments of the world have then tried to develop systems that create an element of "free" care while rigorously dividing the elements of care into packets that move payments for the care over to insurance companies. Along with this, and perhaps more easily, they will simply deny payment on the basis that payment is either limited or not covered for any specific diagnosis. At the same time, in the United States, insurance companies create such policies such as "*if Medicare doesn't cover it, we don't cover it either*." This spares the insurance companies of the burden of trying to determine what they will and won't pay for, based on every element they can contrive. These elements range from defined "pre-existing" considerations to an endless stream of other mandates in their policies, always ending with the final conclusion that denial of payment is assured if Medicare won't cover a claim. Insurance companies essentially default to the government's restrictive policies; in today's computer world, this denial of payment has become almost ridiculously easy. The logic behind the insurance companies' refusing to cover a patient's "pre-existing" conditions rests on the extraordinary cost of health insurance if people were to simply buy their policies only when they get sick. This is, of course, not a process of buying insurance; it is a process of buying care. Most healthy patients are inclined to believe they won't "get sick" and are therefore inclined to *not* purchase insurance when they don't seem to need it; they are essentially playing the odds that they won't get sick and they usually win (until they do get sick). The questions about a "mandate" to buy Obamacare insurance in the United States, and the cancellation of that mandate, was what led to ever-increasing "insurance" costs; the people purchasing this coverage regularly had "pre-existing" conditions—if one waits until he or she gets sick before buying into the plan, a pre-existing condition is assured and the premium cost will skyrocket. A comparison of this process might be that if homeowners wait to buy fire insurance only after their homes are *actually on fire*, the cost predictably will be astronomical.

Which leaves the question with each and every patient who may need medical care or who would like to have medical care made available—who will pay for care? The governments that promote "free" medical care that covers *all* conditions, even the pre-existing ones, will have patients pay significantly higher taxation costs, especially since there is no governmental exclusion (pre-existing or otherwise) for these kinds of treatments. Medicare doesn't have a "pre-existing" exclusion. However, from the government's perspective, this is no problem; simply reduce how much the doctors and the hospitals get paid for Medicare services while increasing taxes. This reduction or denial of payment combined with increasing the taxation of the working population is the source of allowing payment for treatment that is promoted as "free," while stimulating the false political promise of virtually 'free" Medicare for all.

And, while the doctors cannot stay true to the Hippocratic Oath for their patients because of overloaded waiting rooms, overloaded waiting lists, and telephones that ring continuously, at what point would any rational human being simply hang up his or her stethoscope and decide to bale out of the nightmare that has been created and either join a rent-a-doc clinic, or to just simply abandon entirely the practice of primary care medicine?

Chapter 7

The Doctor

Why would anybody in his or her right mind ever want to become a doctor?

Most young people who might become future doctors are intelligent and have a natural aversion to suffering. And when there is a *predictable* high degree of educational intensity extending for years during the preparation for medical school, and for several years thereafter, anybody who has considered a career in medicine must either be unaware of the magnitude of the challenge or must consider the goal to be worth the agony.

The experience of labor begins early in the premedical years, with the college challenges of such courses as calculus, physics, biology, quantitative analysis and organic chemistry, combined with the certainty that, if grades in those classes are not almost exclusively A's, the dream will rapidly fade and the probability of becoming a physician may often also begin to fade. For the high-GPA students, the suffering then becomes magnified during the tortuous time of applying to medical school, usually during the senior year of college. This is a time when most rational human beings must look away from the sheer mass of competitive hopefuls (among the most competitive, 11,417 applicants recently applied to attend UCLA's David Geffen School of Medicine with a class of 184 students).[215] Furthermore, he or she must accept the rigorous requirements to achieve a stellar score on the predictive MCAT (Medical College Admission Test), and must have accumulated an almost perfect Grade Point Average (premed GPA of medical students is 3.93 at top-ranked Johns Hopkins).[216] The hopeful student must also ignore the enormous financial challenge that often stretches at least another decade into the future, finishing with virtually labor-level earnings during the intern and residency learning process.

For a successful outcome, therefore, the future doctor must continuously focus on the *goal*, and it must be something more, much more, than just the excitement of being able to tell friends and family, "I'm going to be a doctor." Finally, if acceptance miraculously occurs and the medical school years are survived, there is the often brutal internship year (a time when one of my UCLA classmates became overwhelmed and committed suicide). And then there are the residency years where the continuing long hours and minimal pay forces the evolving physicians to stay focused on the final goal while trying to start paying off the costs from the many years of education and living expenses. Then, at the end of all that, for most doctors, there is a final rigorous requirement of taking a ten-hour Board Certification examination with hundreds of incredibly challenging questions that have to be answered correctly to become the golden physician who is finally "Board Certified," rather than a more diminutive "Board Eligible" doctor.

And so, with all of this challenge, what exactly is the goal of a career in medicine? For most of us, it would be to apply what we have learned to save or improve a human life, or many human lives...something that most people are *never* able to say they have done throughout their lifetime. Furthermore, the goal is to reduce human suffering, to live a valuable life, to become skilled at treating or curing illness, to prevent disease, and to have gathered so much knowledge and experience as to *really make a difference* for so many patients during the years of a medical career. Such a powerful and complex goal this must be, for the doctors graduating from United States' medical schools, a goal that drives them to continue on during the professional years of practice in spite of the risks from regular exposure to contagious diseases from their patients, in spite of the powerful and personal emotional toll of helplessly watching a suffering patient die, and in spite of the often crushing debt incurred in the process of just getting there. And, most significant is a full understanding of the prelude to the career in medicine, delivered at the end of medical school classroom training, enshrined by speaking the Hippocratic Oath (or some close variant of it) upon graduation, the oath that defines the moral essence of it all.

Yet, not more than 22 years after finishing my training and graduating from medical school, after completing a grinding internship and residency, after passing my board certification examination, after paying off all my debts, and after so many years of helping patients combat the challenges of their diseases, I decided to quit.

This enormous decision came to me unexpectedly as a shock on a Sunday morning as I started a vacation for a week away from my practice while another internal medicine physician covered the medical needs of my patients. In the beginning of my years of my primary care internal medicine practice, I had thrived quickly and the fulfillment of providing patient care was immensely satisfying. My patients loved how I cared for them, and I loved doing it…my practice could not have been more perfect. The time of caring for my patients rapidly became busy, but as the years passed and after I had achieved a satisfying census of about 1,000 patients, increasing elements of stress and financial challenge began to emerge from multiple factors.

My income during those early years and the GI Bill had paid off my medical school and residency training debts, but as the years passed, it became necessary to increase my volume of patients to adjust to progressively declining payment from patients' insurance systems and from the government's Medicare program. This increased volume naturally threatened to create a deterioration in the quality of the care I could deliver to my patients since there was a limit on how many patients could be scheduled and how many hours I could practice each day.

This onerous developing change was insidious. Running my office, there was the expense of the salary and health insurance plans for my office manager and medical assistants, there was the cost of my office rent, the expenses for the computer systems and the medical equipment such as the treadmill, an EKG machine, the examining tables, the pulmonary function testing equipment, sigmoidoscopy equipment, and the cupboards filled with sterile gloves, syringes and needles. On top of these expenses, my mandatory malpractice insurance was expensive (although I have never been sued), and the cost of the transcribing services that allowed for a crisp typed medical record added to the burden of office expenses. These costs continued to climb, and then as increased patient volume became necessary, I needed to add an additional medical assistant.

In response to these increasing costs, I had to begin slowly increasing the fees I charged my patients, and for a time, everything remained stable. My patient load had been manageable, allowing enough time to see each of the patients and to take proper care of them as I declined many requests to further expand my practice. I regularly and routinely made house calls when my patients requested, I answered my patients' calls throughout the night and on weekends as needed. I came to the hospital and took care of my patients whenever they had to visit the emergency room, and I made valuable but time-consuming rounds on my hospitalized patients as I coordinated specialty needs and as I supervised the input from surgeons or other highly trained specialists.

It had seemed important to not further increase my volume of total patients since this would inevitably further diminish the time I could have available for each patient.

And then, the sources of income (that had been the previously reliable direct patient or insurance payments) began to change the entire financial picture. Most of my older patients were covered by the Medicare system, but as computers became more sophisticated, the computer links to my charges for patient care increasingly resulted in a denial of payment if a diagnosis code (using the mandatory so-called "ICD-9 coding" of that time) did not precisely conform to a complex Medicare code, many of them unknown to the physician, difficult to find, or not well explained. Even worse, the medical insurance companies followed this denial pattern, routinely refusing payment for anything that was declined by Medicare—this denial was always explained by the statement: "*Charges disallowed by Medicare are not paid by Secondary Insurance*." These charges then needed to be routinely transferred to the patient who simultaneously was having to pay exorbitant health insurance premiums as the insurance company refused to pay.

As the non-payments for care in my practice became frequent and challenging, I was forced to take on the additional expense of hiring a medical billing company that added its expertise to request payments that were denied. Even with this added professional payment help, the denials of payment continued to climb. As the billing company began to consume increasing amounts of my rapidly declining income, and as the Medicare/insurance payment system continued to send me ever-more notices of denied payment, I was again forced to add even more patients in an effort to cover losses from all the payments not being made while costs continued to spiral up and out of control. Within the next couple of years, my patient census climbed to 2,000 patients, and then a year later to 3,000 patients as Medicare continued to deny or reduce payments for the care I was providing. Inevitably with double and then triple the number of patients, the time available for the care of each patient became shorter, and my risks of making a mistake or missing a diagnosis became greater. And so, it became difficult to find time on my schedule for people who suddenly became ill, or to make time to properly discuss health matters for the new patients with an increased number of medical problems. It also became difficult to squeeze in house calls and to make decent medical rounds on my hospitalized patients.

I looked at the question of hiring one or more Physician Assistants (PAs) to spread the workload, and I considered what these talented people might do to relieve the burden that was becoming overwhelming. I had become aware that the issue of overwhelmed doctors was being addressed by bringing non-MDs up to the front lines by expanding the use of PAs, and other ancillary medical personnel. Yet, for PAs, who have a shorter training time

(26 months compared to at least 7 years for MDs), I questioned whether it would be possible to bring PAs into a primary patient care practice without physician oversight as implied by their title?

Meanwhile, on the main internet information pages for PAs, the presumption is made that they could be some of the answer to the physician shortage: The PAs are educated in intense educational programs lasting a couple of years.... This relatively short training period means that PAs can quickly begin practice, helping offset the worsening physician shortages. It makes good sense that a well-trained PA is invaluable for patient care, and the PA presence does allow a medical doctor more time for better care of additional patients or patients with more complex medical problems. And, it was apparent that, in the setting of specialty care, a PA working in coordination with a specialist medical doctor would indeed help offset the problems of the worsening physician shortages. Furthermore, in even more highly specialized medical settings, an experienced and well-trained PA can have a precise (although limited) knowledge base, much higher than most MDs outside that specialty setting, and may therefore be useful to allowing a doctor to be less restrictive with his or her patient volume.

But would this help work in a primary care office?

A further matter, not so easily identified, is how many patients needing to see a doctor will be told by a managed care receptionist on the telephone that "The PA can see you today but the doctor can see you in a week." Actually, it has been reported[217] that, in this country, 60% of patients must wait 2 weeks for a primary care physician appointment, 20% of patients must wait 4 weeks, and only 10% can see their regular doctor the same day they need care. If there is no alternative choice other than to go to an emergency room, the patient will likely agree for a PA to see him or her. If there is an obscure physical finding that was not a part of this PAs shorter training time, a diagnosis could be delayed, much as it could be for a doctor who is overloaded with patients and stressed for time. It is perhaps best said by the AMA Journal of Ethics that PAs will be increasingly used in primary care, noting their versatility and being "cost-effective clinicians, extending the services of physician practices and improving delivery of care to underserved populations."[218]

It would seem likely that this addition could improve the delivery of care to a patient population defined by the AMA to be "underserved."

But at the same time, the government and Medicare have already initiated the practice of redefining doctors. Starting several years ago, as I have noted, both Medicare and medical insurance companies began calling doctors "Providers"—a term that did not differentiate us from Nurse Practitioners, Physician Assistants, Physical Therapists or Massage Therapists. In my billing returns, I received a "provider" payment notice from Medicare that said the charge for a "Comprehensive Wellness Visit" service was: *"Amount 'Provider' charged= $140, Amount Approved = $0.00,"* and an explanation followed: "This service is Not Approved." The care for the patient had included treatment for multiple conditions and the service was still "Not Approved." Somehow, an hour of professional services by a medical doctor "provider" was not approved.

I looked over their response to my bill, trying to understand how they could do this...during this comprehensive visit, I had done the work, I had helped the patient, I had spent the time and provided my medical expertise to multiple problems but, somehow, it was "Not Approved." I guessed that this related to an ICD-9 diagnosis that was deemed by their computers to be incompatible with the service. This, of course, also meant the insurance company would pay nothing. And so, while I resubmitted inquiries to my expensive billing company, and asked them to try and make the codes work for the comprehensive medical exam, the patient would complain (justifiably) about no Medicare/Insurance payments for his care and asking why he is now being charged for this service. The patient also noted that he, at the same time, had to pay ever-increasing premiums for his "insurance coverage" that followed Medicare, the same insurance company that had refused to pay for his examination even after he had paid hundreds of dollars for his insurance coverage. All of this was, of course, turned over to my billing company who, in turn, increased their charges to me for the added work as they searched for better ICD-9 codes.

For a second, and often recurring, example I discovered that if a billing for an "Established Patient

Office Visit" was somehow approved, the charged amount of $122.58 produced a Medicare statement that said, "'Medicare approved amount' is $81.52" with an explanatory note, "The amount Medicare paid for physician services was reduced due to Federal, State, and local rules." There was no information as to what the "Federal, State, and local rules" might be, the payment was simply reduced by nearly 40% as these unknown "rules" were applied. Furthermore, the insurance companies seemed to be making money from all this as they collected premiums while paying out a lower "insurance coverage."

In the meantime, various government representatives proclaimed publically that they were attentive to the politically inspired mandate of seeking to have "providers" deliver "free care" and, meanwhile, candidates running for office began announcing that, if they could get elected, *free Medicare for all* would become the solution to America's healthcare crisis. There was no mention of the reduced quality of this "free" care.

The result of all this was on that otherwise beautiful Sunday morning, the time arrived for me to quit the practice of medicine. As I tried to reconcile how such moral mandates like those from Hippocrates, would allow a practice to be *"In purity and according to divine law"* which would allow me to *"carry out my life and my art."* I was beginning to feel that, while I was trying to climb the mountain to the Hippocratic Alter of Medicine, I was instead groveling in the mud and engaged in a continuous battle with ICD codes, Medicare, and the insurance industry at the bottom of the cliff.

Also, at that time, my wife (who had worked as a teacher to put me through medical school, and who then worked for years transcribing all the medical records in my office) and my two children, who were in school and trying to live normal lives, found themselves living in the home of a father-doctor who was becoming more and more stressed. I was getting squeezed by the government payment system, squeezed by the insurance payment system, squeezed by patients who wanted (and deserved) more time with their doctor, and I was rapidly reaching the point where, *no matter how many patients I scheduled*, I would not be able to cover the costs after the broad denial of payment for my otherwise thriving primary care medical practice.

There were many reasons finding a doctor for primary care had become difficult. The Covid threat in 2020, carrying on to 2021 and beyond with the expanding Covid variants, had worsened everything for doctors and patients alike, as Zoom office visits prevented examinations of the patient's heart, neurological system, the lungs and the lymph nodes, *and virtually everything important for a decent medical examination*. The potential for diagnostic mistakes with patient diagnoses became greater as physical examinations became impossible. Also, at the same time, Covid-related unemployment created increased issues for patients, with depression, obesity, substance abuse (especially alcohol), while eliminating medical insurance for many patients, forcing them into the burgeoning Medicaid system for their doctor's reimbursement; the number of Medicaid patients in 2010 was about 55 million,[219] climbing to 75 million by 2021. Unfortunately, Medicaid further reduced payments to doctors by around 50% of the usual office charges, meaning that *twice* as many patients must be seen by a doctor per hour just to pay for all the expenses, not counting the expense of the additional Covid mandates such as the cleaning of rooms and equipment between any actual physical examination that might occur. Not surprisingly, it was reported in 2019[220] that less than 68% of primary care doctors will even agree to work within the Medicaid system.

Even more remarkable, during this same time, documented in just one state (California), large numbers of doctors were being scrutinized by the State Medical Board with accusations filed and investigations initiated, resulting in public reprimand, licenses surrendered, licenses revoked, "cease practice" orders, and others. A public record of these California actions (*totaling 1,126 in 2018)* is regularly published and available throughout each year on the internet site www.mbc.ca.gov/Publications/Disciplinary_Actions/ that lists each accused doctor by name, license number and the doctor's city in California. Many of the listed doctors each year are ordered to "surrender" their medical licenses. This number of doctors in 2018 was, remarkably, more than the total of 1,092 *new medical doctors graduating from all California's medical schools that same year.*[221] This happens every single year, over and over, with more than 10,000 doctors' licenses threatened, removed, surrendered, or adversely affected this past decade. If doctors in this one state coming under this attack each year are numerically more than the total annual number of new doctors produced by the medical schools in this state, what does this say about the future of medicine and the availability of doctors to take care of patients?

And then, to make matters even worse, if that is possible, these disciplinary actions are *on top of* the numbers of doctors who are naturally retiring, or being forced into managed care systems, the veteran good doctors who are growing older and becoming tired of the battles inherent with private practices. About 1/3 of all doctors in the United States will be older than 65 in the next ten years[222] and as we have seen, the pressures are becoming intense to retire. It has been estimated by the Association of American Medical Colleges that as many as 55,000 more primary care physicians will naturally retire by 2032 in the United States.

I wondered briefly if organized medicine might help with our worsening circumstances and then I recalled that it has been almost a tradition for doctors to organize poorly, often it is said that medical doctors organize about as well as cats. However, the pattern of declining enrollment in organized medicine is more complicated. The AMA, as previously noted, had dropped in membership from 75% of all American doctors down to 25% (and much less if you discount the number of "doctors in training" and not yet in practice, identified as "members") in the past 50 years. This decimation of AMA membership is seen by many as a disgraceful diminishment from the organization's previous prestigious physician representation since its founding in 1857. In the meantime, the AMA continues to publically promote that it "speaks for doctors" as its membership rolls whither, and remarkably at the same time, it collects substantial sums from the government to provide Medicare "payment coding" by providing the CPT (Current Procedural Terminology). This income source for the AMA, reports medical, surgical, and diagnostic procedures to Medicare and insurance companies; the codes are a registered trademark of the AMA[223] and are paid for and managed by the government entity known as The Centers for Medicare and Medicaid Services (CMS).

How much does the AMA profit from this CPT activity? The organization received in the recent past a revenue of $72 million from "royalties and credentialing products" in association with their government-granted CPT monopoly that sets the fee schedule for Medicare payments.[224] This seems almost outrageous...an organization that claims it represents physicians actually collects twice as much money *from the government* to set doctor payment levels (CPT) than it collects in dues from physician members. This amount of money pouring into the AMA (compared to the relatively paltry $38 million in 2010 member dues) helps validate the widespread assumption that the AMA seems to be more a tool of the government than an organization representing individual physicians trying to practice medicine. And, the most deplorable result of this AMA diminishment is that there is now no representative organization for American doctors to take a stand against the barrage of adverse policies, both in business and from the government and political spectrum that diminishes decent primary care.

And so, as there seemed to be no help from organized medicine, I discovered that more and more doctors are leaving their private practices and migrating into managed care scenarios. It was reported in 2019[225] that 47.4 percent of all doctors had become *employed* physicians (by such behemoth organizations as Kaiser Permanente) while the share of self-employed doctors fell to 45.9 percent. The employed doctors, working in managed care offices, often have large areas of their buildings filled with billing clerks who manage the incomprehensible financial picture. In the meantime, these companies' hired doctors take a reduced salary and endure close monitoring of the amount of time spent per patient and the number of patients seen per hour. The act of hiring these physicians is another confirmation that the bottom (financial) line of a medical practice is important, and in the meantime, the walls around the offices of organized medicine do not often carry versions of the Hippocratic Oath.

And so, finally, as physicians become overwhelmed by billing code denials and increasing expenses, additional doctors who are leaving their private practices have started working for hospitals or hospital-owned facilities.[226] This percent of physicians entering hospital employment has increased from 29% of all doctors in 2012 to nearly 35% of doctors in the past several years. A discerning reader might wonder at this time what happens in smaller communities without managed care complexes, without hiring hospitals, without huge clinics, and without any doctors left who have resisted the overwhelming challenges of trying to continue the practice of medicine. It is apparent that, as this trend continues, the *disappearing doctor,* especially in more rural towns, is becoming a harsh reality for ever-larger numbers of patients.

With all these doctors disappearing from our country's medical landscape, what about *foreign trained* physicians to fill in the doctor-shortage gaps, like they've been trying to accomplish in Canada? In a comprehensive and remarkable review[227] of the volume of foreign trained doctors in this country, it has been noted that currently nearly a *third* of all United States physicians are actually born *outside* the country, and that most of these physicians come from Asia. Also, it has been noted[228] that about 7% of U.S. physicians are currently not even citizens of this country. This can be a positive force, however, for the treatment of patients who have relocated from other countries since, for example, a Chinese trained doctor would have "insider's knowledge" about some of the unique beliefs and methodologies from his or her native country, an asset when bringing healthcare to foreign patients in this country. The Chinese population in some of our larger cities *covet* the finding of a Chinese-trained doctor because, in so many ways, he or she speaks the language.

A review of doctors having complaints launched against them in California (as previously noted to be documented by California's Medical Board) demonstrates many names of foreign nationals among the list but a breakdown of the relative numbers of accusations and investigations against foreign doctors vs. United States trained physicians is not readily available. Primary care doctors are especially affected by this trend, compared to specialty MDs. For example, more than 90% of ophthalmologists, dermatologists, and orthopedic physicians are trained in the United States, while only 61%

of internal medicine physicians are American trained.[229] The trends are clear, however, that as the American population continues to increase and the number of medical schools remains stagnant, increasing numbers of doctors leave the primary care arena.

It has become apparent on so many levels that an American patient's ability to find a doctor will continue to become ever more challenging. And that brings us back to my decision to quit the practice of medicine.

About an hour into my Sunday morning walk, I began to firm up the consideration that I would definitely have to quit and that the time had come to do *anything else* that allowed financial survival. At the same time, I also felt committed to doing *anything* to help ensure my patients would be able to find a new physician by my personal referrals.

And, that was the moment that I had an epiphany.

There was really no problem with my practice of medicine. I woke up each morning enthusiastic about fixing the myriad of issues that caused suffering in my patients' lives, I enjoyed jumping into my car and racing off to the hospital or making a house call or two with my medical assistant, and I enjoyed the inspiration and insightful discussions with my patients during their comprehensive physical exams. We had a superb hospital nearby, within walking distance from my office, with outstanding nurses who worked with me to stabilize and cure the patients I had to admit. And, since my patients seemed to appreciate what I was doing, there was no problem with the fundamental elements of my working through each day (and often through the night) as their personal physician.

At the same time, I had no interest in following so many primary care physicians out of private practice and into a clinic, to become a hired doc working for a manager or a company instead of for my patients. Although I was a six-year veteran of the U.S. Navy, I had little desire to begin working for the government at our local VA hospital. Most important, I never wanted to work in a setting where clusters of non-MD management people would tell me how many patients I had to see each hour, how much time I could spend with each patient, and how many other physician's practices I would regularly have to cover. I knew many doctors were moving in that direction, or in the direction of a hiring hospital, and were doing so for the many reasons, the most important being to escape the billing challenges and all the associated paperwork issues I had been regularly facing.

I simply felt those medical practice settings were not for me.

So.... If the problem is not the patients, and the problem is not my training or the process of caring for sick patients, what is left? My whole career, from the premedical study days through medical school and residency has been related to patient care and that element was a continuing professional pleasure. And so, the answer emerged that, since the government and insurance companies now control so much of patient care and doctor's lives, what would my patients say to the concept of taking care of them *without billing for each service and without involving Medicare or insurance companies*? Is it possible to just take care of patients without these entities? And, at the same time, could I then discontinue my relationship with the billing service that had become so necessary to challenge the Medicare and insurance denials?

Would it be possible to just say goodbye to the government and to the insurance companies, to them all...but ***not*** *to my patients?*

Would it be possible to become a physician again and not a "service provider?" Would the patients still want to see me as their physician? It seemed obvious that, at least within the realm of primary care, since the patients had been virtually removed from the payment system already by Medicare and insurance companies, why wouldn't those patients be happy to continue with a physician who also eliminated third-party payment systems, *especially if he didn't charge the patient for each element of care*? Finally, since I could trim the volume of patient overload, and I would therefore have more time to take care of individual patients, to see patients more quickly without any overload delay or the tremendous morass of billing issues, couldn't I provide even better care? If I took this action, which nobody in our city had ever done, wouldn't I become a better doctor?

But...how would the patients then cover the costs of my practice of medicine?

Would they be willing to occasionally send me a payment, maybe, *once per year*...a "prepayment" of sorts for my availability throughout the year to provide all of their primary medical care, without any further billing? Would it work if everybody had exactly the same charge, rich or financially struggling, old or young, healthy or sick? And, if I could also just send a personalized letter to each patient once per year for a renewal prepayment request for each of them to remain in my new practice...would anybody actually continue? Furthermore, how many patients would even *want* to join? There was no previous experience in our small community of any doctor doing that, could it work? Is it legal? Finally, if I eliminated all the government/insurance/billing costs from my practice how much should I charge each patient for joining a practice with a smaller number of patients, perhaps a *much* smaller number?

It seemed immediately apparent that the process of making such a change could actually be remarkably simple. To allow the maximum amount of time for patient visits without any rushing, to allow the continuation of the occasional house call or emergency room visit, to allow scheduling of patients *that same day* when problems emerged in their lives, to have a practice without a waiting room jammed with sick patients waiting forever, sounded great but how many patients should I have in my practice?

I already knew that having 3,000 patients under my care was vastly too many to allow the kind of quality care I wanted to provide.... But, how many fewer would be appropriate? Maybe a total of 500, or even perhaps 300? Could that work, and if it did, how much would I need to charge on an annual basis? Clearly, the fewer patients I saw, the greater the annual cost per patient, while the more patients I saw, the lower the cost but, at some point, also the lower the quality of care...somewhere in the middle of all that would be a perfect number.

There have been many stories of physicians who became "VIP" doctors, serving tiny numbers of "VIP" patients for vast sums of money. Elvis Presley's and Jerry Lee Lewis' doctor, and Michael Jackson's doctor came to mind, and I recalled that both doctors developed massive legal problems and lost their licenses to practice medicine. And I was quite certain that taking care of a very small number of VIP's would not be satisfying, since these "important people" would be paying large amounts while instructing the doctor, like a hired hand, what they wanted, when they wanted it, and how you would have to comply. You would become more of a servant than a physician; because of their VIP fame, you would be at their "beck and call," and doing what they tell you to do rather than necessarily doing the right thing and providing the best possible care.

Also, this would not follow any of Hippocrates' moral guidance and it would not be what *real* doctors should do.

So, taking care of 1 or 2 patients was ridiculous, taking care of 3,000 was a nightmare. Again, what about several hundred patients, maybe 200 or 300? Would they be willing to pay me for my care, would I be able to give them superb care, could it work, *would* it work? If 300 patients was the maximum volume of this newly imagined practice, what about the upper end of the *volume* issue and what about the compelling moral argument that doctors should never exclude any patients at any time?

It is believed by some that doctors should be humanitarians who had a moral obligation to take care of *all* patients who come to their office door seeking help. But, if I were to follow that philosophy, even with the best of humanitarian motivations, the result would inevitably be the same kind of deteriorated care I had been experiencing as I tried to help 3,000 patients. I had already learned that, past a certain point, the higher the volume, the greater the deterioration of the care for all of the patients...that would be a compelling humanitarian argument *against* seeing "all patients who knock on the office door." It seemed possible that as many as 4,000 or 5,000 patients might desire my care if I opened the doors without restrictions...however, could I ever deliver quality medical services to that number of patients, could I even find room on the schedule for them, and would it be possible to spend more than 5 minutes or so in a rushed visit as I tried to hear their problems and examine their bodies? Within the medical profession, stories abound about rushed physicians, often within an HMO setting and while in the room with a patient, hearing the knocking of the door as a staff announces that the next patient is waiting. Wrap up your exam, doctor, move the patient out, you have *another* patient waiting.

Wouldn't I become like just another HMO, hoping I could retire before going crazy?

Clearly, there would have to be a line beyond which I would regretfully have to turn patients away, a point where I would have to tell prospective new patients that "I'm sorry, my practice is full," no matter how difficult that might be. It was also clear that, looking at the national picture and considering the challenges those turned-away patients faced in finding a doctor, there would have to be, for society, a vigorous effort to produce more doctors in our country, especially in primary care. Is it even politically possible to create an urgent mandate for a country needing more doctors, perhaps initiating a war-like directive to produce additional primary care doctors by creating additional medical schools, maybe enlarge some of the classes in the current schools, and perhaps consider medical training programs that focus on fixing the depleted ranks of primary care doctors? Would it be possible to create financial incentives to eliminate the school costs to medical students who fulfill a mandate of specializing in primary care? Hasn't this become a national need, and if so, shouldn't there be a national program initiated to answer the need? Considering all the millions of dollars pouring into wasteful political agendas, couldn't some of this be directed into an aggressive effort to train more primary care doctors?

I had also been aware of a couple of physicians, including former Seattle SuperSonics physician, Dr. Howard Maron, and Dr. Scott hall in Seattle, who had been practicing in a so-called "concierge" clinic practice called MD2, for an annual fee."[230] That early startup has, over the years, been expanded now to the Virginia Mason Hospital and clinics, featuring an extremely user-friendly website and listing numerous concierge physicians available for care.[231] My charge to my patients would be somewhere close to what their system charged, I suspected, in anticipation of my discarding the billing company expenses as well as those who generated the "denial of payment" notifications from the government and insurance companies.

Another concierge care physician group in America is a company founded in 2000 in Boca Raton, Florida called MDVIP, with about 700 employees and an annual revenue of $400,000,000.[232] The name of this company implies that each patient (or doctor?) has some VIP royalty blood...not the kind of message I envisioned where my patients would be just good people I would enjoy carrying for. Also, they promote that they would limit each doctor's number of patients to "no more than 600 patients," with an average annual cost of $1800,[233] although their current website advertises, "the annual fee for MDVIP-affiliated practices ranges between $1,650 and $2,200" per year.[234] This system continues to sign up doctors around the country, and their current website advertises their doctors "practice medicine the way they were trained," also noting the MDVIP company will bill Medicare and insurance companies for the additional funds they would be able to collect.[235] They state that their doctors "want to maintain their independence" although it was not clear to me how they are "independent" while linked to such a national MDVIP organization that is, furthermore, linked with the primary problem of Medicare billing issues and insurance companies. It would also be helpful to know how much of this patient-generated income is diverted into the advertising dollars that are seen across the country. Finally, their website is filled with *testimonials* from doctors and patients...I had always considered the testimonial element of advertising to be a dark stain on physicians' reputations.

Other competing concierge systems include companies with such names as Concierge Choice Physicians, Elite Health, and Signature MD, were firms reported to have annual revenues ranging from $10,000,000 to $15,000,000.[236] The websites that promote and advertise these companies are professional and glitzy, showing beautiful and healthy-appearing patients, caring and compassionate-appearing physicians, and they streamline the process of "applying" for both doctors and patients. They uniformly tout the advantages of the concierge model, and they do appear to avoid testimonials that could create the sense of hucksterism and excessive self-promotion. Price comparisons between the different organizations, and service comparisons can be challenging for patients and doctors, although an effort is made to find a "local" member physician for patients in a number of different states. The "annual revenue" numbers for these companies should be a clear reminder that the companies have financial agreements with physicians, with patients, with Medicare, and possibly with insurance companies which again takes us all back to the challenges of either denied service or denied payment for services outside an uncertain sphere of defined care.

If my "concierge" concept were to *remove* outside billing agencies and outside sources of payments, why would I want to join a system that *uses* these government and private agencies? And, why would I want to *pay* a company to do that? I would not want to advertise and I would not want to pay a concierge company to advertise for me...word-of-mouth has always been the best mechanism for obtaining new patients. And, from the patient's perspective, the biggest challenge is the same challenge for any social media or Web media definition for excellence—the computer screen can show or tell a perspective patient anything a marketing company can generate to speak convincingly of compassionate quality care. But the gold standard for physician selection should always be "word-of-mouth," the comments and recommendations from those who have received care from any specific doctor who practices nearby. The best "word-of-mouth" is often from another physician in the community, or frequently from a nurse in the area, either of whom could recommend a doctor with a basis of insider knowledge about that doctor's level of expertise in the care of patients.

It became apparent that, since I first considered this change in my practice, (with the complete quitting of medicine as my alternative), there has been a progressive acceleration in the number of doctors following this "concierge" model. According to a national trade magazine, Concierge Medicine Today, out of the nearly 221,000 primary care medical doctors in the United States, approximately 12,000 doctors (mostly primary care internists or family practitioners) have abandoned the onerous "fee-for-service" model and have become concierge physicians. It is challenging to determine how many of these doctors have taken this action on their own rather than by signing up with (and paying for) a national organization, but considering how successful it can be for the patient and the doctor, there should be a high number of doctors doing this on their own.

These 12,000 doctors who have escaped the government and insurance mandates are a small percent of American doctors, but their numbers are estimated to be growing by 3-6% per year. The general business pattern for these concierge doctors spreads fees over a wide range, somewhat dependent on how many patients the doctor has in his or her practice. The average cost to patients appears to average between $125 and $150 per month, or about $2,000 per year (although sometimes much more). And notably, there are a number of other concierge practices with doctors who charge huge sums for a tiny number of patients; this group included physicians in the Beverly Hills area, or other wealthy areas in larger cities where patients were offered deluxe concierge services, super-VIP services, for annual fees as much as $7,000 or more per person, occasionally even much more. That seemed like a unnecessarily large annual fee unless the doctor is seeing a very tiny number of patients, like those MDs who limited their practice to the wealthy and/or famous. Again, these kinds of practices shift the emphasis from providing great care over to collecting great amounts of money while becoming less of a physician and more of a servant to the rich and famous.

Finally, returning as always to the Hippocratic Oath, there were no considerations from this Father of Medicine for providing anything other than quality care with a high degree of ethics and morality.

And so, I wondered if it would be possible for any individual doctor to just quietly, without input or financial support from any organizations like MDVIP, or like Seattle's MD2, or the Virginia Mason system and the others, to simply morph his or her practice into a prepaid system without any advertisements or testimonials? Would it be possible for this physician to offer a practice asking for a single payment each year, or even a prepayment each month?

Also, at the very beginning, I made the unique decision to not bill *anybody* besides the single annual billing to the patient. I would simply keep track of each patient's annual payment through a Microsoft Word and Microsoft Excel document on my home computer—it would not add to my practice costs, it would be simple, once per year for each patient, and it should keep me up to date about when a future personalized renewal letter would be sent to a patient each year. And, I would more easily be able to provide the highest level of *individual patient care* possible.

Two weeks later, as the decision was finalized, I sent 2,700 letters to my existing patients telling them I could no longer continue in my existing practice, and I reassured them that my office staff would do everything possible to help them find a new doctor during the transition. Also, I reassured them I would continue to care for them for the next several months until they could find a new doctor and I would help them as much as possible in that effort.

At the same time, in the same mailbox, I mailed an additional 300 letters to the patients I had cared for the longest, the people to whom I had grown most attached, and individuals with a wide range of financial standings. I invited these people to join my new practice for a single annual fee that would hopefully be manageable. Also, I told them in this letter that, for a small additional fee, I would include their children who had grown beyond the pediatric age in the practice. Finally, I informed them that, if they joined, there would be no additional billings during each year for any care I would provide and I told them this annual fee would remain unchanged for the rest of their lives. I outlined the care they would receive, the whole usual spectrum that included my availability for regular routine office visits (the scheduling of ½ hour for patient visits), and I reminded them that I would continue providing careful and attentive annual comprehensive exams. In the letter, I told them I would also be fully available for prompt unscheduled emergency visits to my office if needed, and I would continue to make house calls as they might become necessary. They were assured that I was available for direct cell phone after-hours calls throughout the night for help at any time with any emergencies, without recordings or answering service intrusions, and that they would, if needed, receive the best possible hospital care (either in patient rooms or in the intensive care units). Finally I told them that in my office, they would have available, at no additional charge, EKGs, treadmills, breathing tests, and everything else needed for them to stay healthy.

I said in the letter that I hoped the cost for this would be manageable, (even for those patients with just social security payments as a major source of income), and

I let them know my entire office staff would continue helping with their care as before. My annual charge would be the same for each of my entire spectrum of patients, some of whom were wealthy owners of companies, some who were retired in tiny homes and living off Social Security, a couple of whom owned large boats and travelled around the world, two of whom had won the Nobel Prize in Physics, several good people regularly employed in their daily jobs, and many young patients with growing families that included children.

I advised them that, although I would not have involvement with it, their Medicare linkage and their insurance coverage should continue to cover whatever costs they may incur outside my practice. For example, if a patient needed a mammogram, it would be important to have some financial coverage for such a test; as we have seen, there are huge cost variations for such tests. And, if an emergency evaluation in the hospital setting was needed, if lab tests were needed, if a hospitalization was necessary, or surgery was performed, the Medicare and insurance systems should be helpful to cover the potentially huge charges that may result. Some patients additionally considered changing their insurance coverage to "catastrophic care," a change which lowers their premium costs but increases (sometimes greatly) their up-front deductible charges for hospital or radiologic testing.

Finally, I resolved that this practice would never be called "concierge medicine." The word *concierge* just seems to suggest elements of aristocracy, with regal-like care, like what a king or some kind of royalty might receive, or perhaps what a VIP hotel guest might be offered, seemingly a highbrow or elitist philosophy. In my mind, the care I provided would be because I was trained to be the doctor for the individual who was my patient, not because the individual had a royal position in life. Just the unlimited definition of "concierge" seemed inappropriate to me—in the hotel industry, a "concierge" is somebody who performs services like making reservations, booking transportation, arranging for local visits, recommending sightseeing spots, and coordinating bell desk service etc. A good concierge person could even arrange for excellent theater tickets...not exactly consistent with my profession. Interestingly enough, the ancient meaning of the word, during times of Greek or medieval times, originated from the French phrase "comte des cierges" and describes the person who lit the candles and maintained them at major events. Also, among the many additional translations of "concierge" are a jailor, an escort, a bouncer, and a hired gun....

So, what to call my new practice, should anybody actually consider joining? I considered "Traditional Care" but it was not particularly catchy, and other terms that might include "the best possible medical care from a doctor who cares" seemed weird. Finally, I determined that I did not need a name for my "system" since it coincided with the important elements of traditional care learned in medical school and within that system, I would deliver the kind of attention of which Hippocrates would approve. The only name on my practice, which would have zero marketing, was Roger C. Dunham, M.D. and I hoped that would be good enough for those who traditionally, by word of mouth, had been drawn to my office.

And so I sent the letters, all 3,000 of them, out to my patients and I waited for the response. I thought about the entire scenario again; I was determined that, if this didn't work, that would be the end of my medical career.

Silence followed the mailings...for about two days. Nobody called with anger, nobody called with happiness, and nobody accused me of abandoning them or of not caring about them...nobody called me about *anything.*

And then one of my invited patients, an elderly and sweet 90-year-old patient, slowly entered my medical office's door one afternoon, and using her cane for balance, slowly moved across the waiting area and up to my receptionist's window.

"I would like to join Dr. Dunham's new practice," she said in a weak voice as she pulled out a crumpled check and, with shaking hands, wrote out the annual fee and signed it. My office manager thanked her and let her know she was the first patient to join and that we would all take good care of her.

"I know you will," she said, and added as she turned away, "you always have."

The incoming mail delivery that day included a couple more envelopes of people joining, and the next day there were more. By the end of the week, 20 or more envelopes arrived each day. It took almost a month before nearly everybody who had been sent a letter of invitation joined my practice. During those weeks, as the envelopes poured in, I worked with my staff to find new doctors for my patients who had not been included in the invitation and the process proceeded smoothly. In a little more than a month, my practice had been trimmed down by 2,700 patients, my schedule had changed from 20-25 patients per day to 5 or 6 people each day, my office staff smiled much more and seemed to be happier as my practice began continuously providing the kind of care for which I had been trained, the kind of care envisioned by Hippocrates and the kind of care which regularly fulfilled my dream of my future life as a doctor. And, significantly, my office manager at the front desk would never be compelled to ask, "Did you bring your insurance card?"

I was the first physician in our community to start this new kind of medical practice, and it continued unchanged, allowing me to provide the best possible care for the next 18 years. Most of the local primary care physicians have initiated similar practice patterns and several specialists (primarily in the internal medicine subspecialty ranks) have done the same.

I had made several discoveries upon that initiation and during the years that followed:

- The start-up of the practice was remarkably easy, but did require a pool of patients who would trust me to provide the kind of care I offered. The summary of the payment mechanism was simple: send out personal letters of invitation, together with letters that informed those not invited as I closed my fee-for-service practice. That sending of letters, along with the personalized renewal letters sent each year thereafter, eliminated all the insurance and government challenges as my practice became satisfying and continuously a professional pleasure.
- None of these patients in my single-payment-once-per-year practice created increased visits or calls—they were happy to be in the practice and apparently nobody wanted to jeopardize that relationship.

- There were no legal actions or requirements necessary to complete this change. A brief effort by the insurance industry in my state tried to declare this model of practice to be "insurance," requiring certification by an "insurance commissioner," but that effort disappeared as other doctors throughout our city and the state started the same kind of practice and the loss of physicians by any "cease and desist" order would have been intolerable to the public.
- Income remained stable for nearly two decades, and I was able to keep all the retainer fees unchanged for my original patients during the time that followed. Although no patient in this initial group ever saw an increase in their original costs for my care, and as new patients joined over the years (after existing patients moved or eventually passed on) they were charged slightly more to compensate for inflationary costs of medical assistant salaries, rent, and the costs of equipment. And, these new patients' annual costs then remained the same for those patients for as long as I was their doctor.

- The small number of patients I had who would or did become covered by the Medicaid system for the indigent were seen without charge—this was easily accomplished and their appreciation was fulfilling.
- When I finally retired from a practice with this system in place, I was also able to interview extremely high-quality physicians from the best medical training programs before finally selecting a superb doctor who readily committed to continue the practice as I had established. And, because of this, the patients benefited from compassionate expertise that might not have been available from a new overloaded, overworked, or less qualified doctor.
- Doctors who have tried to follow this pathway, and *who continue to bill insurance and Medicare*, should understand the costs of billing and all the headaches that are part of the denials and the reductions in reimbursement are not worth it—in primary care, these insurance and government payment systems will often continue as an expensive and continuing nightmare.

- Since this kind of practice, *by its nature*, allows the care of fewer patients (even with the help of Physician Assistants), there needs to be a vigorous effort by our elected leaders to stimulate the building of additional medical schools and primary care medical training systems to provide physicians who may care for the patients. As the supply of doctors diminishes, there will be an ever-increasing number of patients seeking help that cannot be provided.

The early days of my medical practice, using fee-for-service as the model for payment and following the guidance of Hippocrates worked well. The patients were happy, the payments were adequate, I had the time to provide care in the manner taught at UCLA, and life within my medical practice was good. As time passed, however, and as the insurance industry began to control the very essence of medicine, complicit with the government in this evolution that became truly an assault and violation of the Hippocratic Oath, the changes forced on patients and doctors became, at best, deplorable. Other medical systems around the world have struggled with similar problems that have made the delivery of care so challenging; from China through Russia, England, and Canada, all have tried to finance something that (as medicine advanced and became more complex and expensive) could allow patients to receive care without bankrupting the individuals and the country.

For all doctors, decisions must be made regarding their patterns of care in each of their offices. Following the Hippocratic Oath, the question must be asked, is it better to see large numbers of patients (with lowered time and less quality-of-care for each patient) or is it better to see a smaller number of patients (with more available time and better quality-of-care for each patient)? It seems clear that the Hippocratic mandate for doctors is to provide the best quality of care for each patient, *and to take the time to do it right.* It is the government's responsibility to expand the training of enough physicians to have the time that allows for the fulfillment of each patient's healthcare needs in our country.

This process can be successful for medical care in a country, as it was for my practice. This can only work, however, if the constraints on primary care doctor training facilities are lifted, and if the medical schools are increased in size and number to produce more of the finest doctors possible. And, I believe, Hippocrates would be satisfied with how patients are treated as his moral mandate begins to experience a renewal, while American medicine becomes sustained as the best in the world.

About the Author

Roger C. Dunham, M.D. is a primary care internal medicine physician with more than 40 years of private practice experience, delivering care to thousands of patients. His medical experience, after graduating from the UCLA School of Medicine in 1975, ranges from caring for the prisoners on the Jail Ward of Los Angeles County Hospital, to caring for patients on the wards of three hospitals in a coastal California community. His unique practice included regularly making house calls as well as caring for patients in intensive care units and in his private office. He has served on several nonprofit Boards of Directors, and as an instrument-rated private pilot has flown many flights of mercy for patients with Angel Flight West. Prior to his medical career, Dr. Dunham served for six years aboard a fast attack nuclear submarine as a reactor operator engaged in espionage activity under the Pacific Ocean. He is the author of several additional books, including Spy Sub (Naval Institute Press), Final Diagnosis (Penguin Press), Rogue Captain, and Surviving Mortality, and he has recently produced a screenplay for the full-length motion picture, Rogue Captain. Dr. Dunham has two children, six grandchildren and has been married to his wife, Keiko, for more than 54 years.

Sources, Appreciation

It has been my good fortune to have the input and advice from several individuals before, during, and after the years of my medical practice. John Dandona and Jim Young provided encouragement and important perspectives about quality factors with my primary care elements, guiding me with concepts of care. Chris and Judith Rose, and Gary Strand gave me perspectives about medicine in the United Kingdom. Alasdair Hilleary provided valuable information about medical care in Scotland, as Val Muth advised me about Canadian care and the challenges of obtaining primary care services as well as Specialty Care. Jill McDowell educated me about important concepts about medicine in Russia based on her own experiences and her book, *Lost in Mother Russia.* Lisa Lu was instrumental in clarifying the complexities of the background of Asian and Chinese medicine, providing input that was invaluable. Locally, Dana Schmitz, working with the David Geffen School of Medicine at UCLA, afforded me with important information relating to the Hippocrates influence at the school and the elements relating to the Hippocratic Oath spoken there by graduating medical doctors. Finally, in our own community, Chen Chin, PharmD, contributed much of his time and wisdom in guiding me through the complexities of pharmaceutical practices and the influence of large systems on the viability of independent drugstores.

[1] Primary Care - Bureau of Health Workforce – HRSAbhw.hrsa.gov › bhw › nchwa › projectingprimarycare
[2] https://calmatters.org/projects/californias-worsening-physician-shortage-doctors/
[3] The Homa Files, Professor Ken Homa, Georgetown University, https://homafiles.info/2017/08/08/how-many-medical-schools-are-there/
[4] Peterson Center on Healthcare, KFF, https://www.healthsystemtracker.org/chart-collection/u-s-health-care-resources-compare-countries/#item-magnetic-resonance-imaging-mri-units-per-million-population-2019
[5] United States Census Bureau
[6] NPR, California Is 1st State To Offer Health Benefits To Adult Undocumented Immigrants, July 10, 2019, Bobby Allyn
[7] ThoughtCo, Top Medical Schools in California, By Allen Grove, Updated July 03, 2019, https://www.thoughtco.com/medical-schools-in-california-4689156#:~:text=Statewide%2C%20only%2012%20California%20universities,schools%20in%20the%20United%20States.
[8] Personal communication, Chinese patient
[9] *Spy Sub*, Roger C. Dunham, Naval Institute Press, 1996
[10] *Surviving Mortality*, Roger C. Dunham, 2017
[11] Wikipedia: Life Expectancy
[12] CDC, MMWR, October 01, 1999 / 48(38);849-858, https://www.cdc.gov/mmwr/preview/mmwrhtml/mm4838a2.htm
[13] America's Health Rankings, United Health Foundation, https://www.americashealthrankings.org/explore/health-of-women-and-children/measure/IMR_MCH/state/ALL
[14] Life in 1907 - Frederick SD Official websitewww.fredericksd.com › life-in-1907
[15] U.S. Life Expectancy 1950-2020 | MacroTrends
[16] NPR: https://www.npr.org/sections/coronavirus-live-updates/2021/07/21/1018590263/u-s-life-expectancy-fell-1-5-years-2020-biggest-drop-since-ww-ii-covid
[17] PNAS: Proceedings of the National Academy of Sciences of the United States of America, https://www.pnas.org/content/118/5/e2014746118
[18] https://www.quora.com/What-would-the-life-span-of-humans-be-

2000-years-ago

[19] Sapiens; Anthropology/Everything Human, Did Ancient People Die Young? Christine Cave, Aug 17, 2018

[20] Dogs' Life Expectancy: buzzle.com/articles/dogs-life-expectancy.html

[21] How long does animals live, Ocean Blue Adventures, oceanadventures.co.za/long-animals-live/

[22] Wildlife, https://www.discoverwildlife.com/animal-facts/...

[23] Science News Shorter men live longer, study shows, May 9, 2014, University of Hawaii at Manoa

[24] Lloyd Brandts, Piet a Van Den Brandt. Body size, non-occupational physical activity and the chance of reaching longevity in men and women: findings from the Netherlands Cohort Study. Journal of Epidemiology & Community Health, 2019 DOI: 10.1136/jech-2018-211410

[25] English Online, https://www.english-online.at/geography/life-expectancy/life-expectancy-where-people-live-longer.htm

[26] AACRAO Edge, https://www.aacrao.org/edge/country/andorra

[27] Which country's people have the longest life expectancy and why? Josh Clark, Copyright © 2020 HowStuffWorks, a division of InfoSpace Holdings, LLC, a System1 Company

[28] Let the dead teach the living" a common expression, calling for autopsies, in the classes of modern medical schools and anatomy courses, first expressed hundreds of years ago in Latin: Mortui vivis praecipiant

[29] The works of Galen are listed in Galenic corpus. https://en.wikipedia.org/wiki/Galen#Contributions_to_medicine

[30] The Criminal and the Saintly Body: Autopsy and Dissection in Renaissance Italy Author(s): Katharine Park Reviewed work(s):Source: Renaissance Quarterly, Vol. 47, No. 1 (Spring, 1994), pp. 1-33, Published by: The University of Chicago Press on behalf of the Renaissance Society of America, Stable URL: http://www.jstor.org/stable/2863109

[31] Autopsy › News in Science (ABC Science), Published 23 October 2002

[32] We demonstrated the remarkable asphyxiation to our anatomy professor—he never did come to believe that we had actually discovered such a bizarre cause of death, but he gave us high grades for our efforts.

[33] Healthline, Medically reviewed by Deborah Weatherspoon, Ph.D., R.N., CRNA — Written by Brian Krans — Updated on August 4, 2017,

https://www.healthline.com/health/heimlich-maneuver

[34] Expansively described by FamilyDoctor.Org (American Academy of Family Physicians) as: Crying for no obvious reason, crying around the same time each day, clenching the fists or curling up the legs crying, crying like you're in pain, and turning bright red when crying.

[35] Sanders L. Every Patient Tells a Story. New York: Broadway Books; 2009:6–91.

[36] Beckman HB, Frankel RM. The effect of physician behavior on the collection of data. Ann Intern Med. 1984;101(5):692–696.

[37] © Copyright 2019 Supervised Visitation Network Worldwide, 2019 California Hospice and Palliative Care Association (CHAPCA)

[38] Ibid

[39] © 2020 Crossroads Hospice, https://www.crossroadshospice.com/hospice-palliative-care-blog/2017/july/13/remembering-dame-cicely-saunders-founder-of-hospice/

[40] Ibid

[41] A human, and therefore capable of mistakes. The phrase emphasizes someone's humanity and fallibility.

[42] Caduceus as a Symbol of Medicine, Wikipedia, the free encyclopedia edited on 31 August 2020. Wikipedia® is a registered trademark of the Wikimedia Foundation, Inc., a non-profit organization.

[43] Florida Healthcare Plans, PELVIC EXAMINATION INFORMED CONSENT, https://www.fhcp.com/documents/10799_U65-0720-Pelvic-Exam-Consent-Form-3.pdf

[44] BCE refers to "Before the Common Era" and is exactly the same numerical value as "B.C." It was changed in modern times to express a sensitivity for those who are not adherents of Christianity, where "Before Christ" might seem offensive. A "C" for "Common," therefore, is numerically exactly the same designation as a "C" for Christ. Furthermore the word "Common" simply indicates the year is based on the most frequently used and common calendar (the Gregorian calendar). It is all superficial verbiage since the numerical values are the same…a Christian can think of Christ, or the birthdate of Christ, while non-Christians can think of Common.

[45] A general of Athens during its golden years, and well-known as a prominent and influential Greek statesman.

[46] Wesley D. Smith, School of Arts and Sciences at the University of Pennsylvania

[47] Wikipediaen.wikipedia.org › wiki › Hippocrates

[48] Margotta, Roberto (1968), The Story of Medicine, New York: Golden Press
[49] The MedLaw Update, The newsletter of the Medical Liability and Health Care Law Committee, 10/15/2018, Volume 23, Issue 2
[50] ibid
[51] Schwartz, Robert A.; Richards, Gregory M.; Goyal, Supriya (2006), Clubbing of the Nails, WebMD, retrieved September 28, 2006
[52] Association of American Physicians and Surgeons, Inc., https://www.aapsonline.org/ethics/oaths.htm
[53] ibid
[54] Written in 1964 by Louis Lasagna, Academic Dean of the School of Medicine at Tufts University, and used in many medical schools today
[55] Adapted from the original by the late Sherman M. Mellinkoff, M.D., Dean, 1962-1986 Professor of Medicine,1962-2016 David Geffen School of Medicine at UCLA
[56] Of the Epidemics.Jun 22, 2020 First, do no harm - Harvard Health Blog - Harvard Health Publishing
www.health.harvard.edu
[57] www.statnews.com 2016
[58] Jun 2, 2017 www.beckersasc.com › leadership ›
[59] ©Peter Tyson, editor in chief of NOVA Online, Created February 2009
[60] ibid
[61] Business Insider, Science Contributors, Judith Graham, STAT Dec 22, 2016
[62] Wall Street Journal, "Doctors, Once GOP Stalwarts, Now More Likely to Be Democrats," By Janet Adamy and Paul Overberg, Oct. 6, 2019
[63] ibid
[64] ibid
[65] Personal conversations at hospital meetings
[66] WSJ Letters to Editor, Rebekah Bernard, M.D., Saturday/Sunday September 26-27, 2020
[67] Adams, Francis (1891), The Genuine Works of Hippocrates, New York: William Wood and Company.
[68] The foundation upon which Western medical practice was built. Also, see: Pavlidis, N.; Karpozilos, A. (2004-09-01). "The treatment of cancer in Greek antiquity." European Journal of Cancer. 40 (14): 2033–2040. doi:10.1016/j.ejca.2004.04.036. ISSN 1879-0852. PMID 15341975.
[69] Tuke, John Batty (1911). "Hippocrates" . In Chisholm, Hugh (ed.).

Encyclopædia Britannica. 13 (11th ed.). Cambridge University Press. pp. 517–519.

[70] https://www.thegreekherbalist.com/herbalcolumn/medicinalherbsinancientgreece

[71] https://www.historyextra.com/period/ancient-history/ancient-drug-use-history-how-what-for-opium-hemp/

[72] https://www.sciencemag.org/news/2019/06/oldest-evidence-marijuana-use-discovered-2500-year-old-cemetery-peaks-western-china

[73] https://www.theatlantic.com/science/archive/2018/04/are-we-earths-only-civilization/557180/

[74] https://en.wikipedia.org/wiki/Human

[75] https://www.sciencemag.org/news/2019/06/oldest-evidence-marijuana-use-discovered-2500-year-old-cemetery-peaks-western-china

[76] ibid

[77] https://www.fda.gov/media/131874/download, FDA at a glance, October, 2019

[78] https://reason.com/2020/04/06/why-you-shouldnt-trust-anyone-who-claims-80-percent-of-americas-drugs-come-from-china/

[79] http://www.pbmwatch.com

[80] Garrison, Fielding H. (1966), History of Medicine, Philadelphia: W.B. Saunders Company

[81] Tuke, John Batty (1911). "Hippocrates". In Chisholm, Hugh (ed.). *Encyclopædia Britannica*. **13** (11th ed.). Cambridge University Press. pp. 517–519.

[82]https://www.ch.ic.ac.uk/rzepa/mim/drugs/html/digitalis.htm#:~:text=Digitalis%20is%20an%20example%20of,since%20its%20discovery%20in%201775.

[83] https://www.gutenberg.org/ebooks/24886

[84] https://www.drugchannels.net/2019/10/the-big-three-wholesalers-revenues-and.html

[85] https://www.drugs.com/article/average-wholesale-price-awp.html

[86] ibid

[87] http://www.pbmwatch.com/dir-fees.html

[88] https://truveris.com/what-is-a-pharmacy-benefit-manager-pbm-and-how-does-a-pbm-impact-the-pharmacy-benefits-ecosystem/

[89] ibid

[90] http://www.pbmwatch.com/pbm-litigation-overview.html

[91]https://www.commonwealthfund.org/publications/explainer/2019/apr/pharmacy-benefit-managers-and-their-role-drug-spending
[92] ibid
[93] https://www.healthline.com/health-news/is-your-doctor-getting-paid-to-prescribe-painkillers-for-you
[94] http://www.ethicaldoctor.org/about-ame/mission-statement/
[95] https://www.cnbc.com/2021/06/07/biogen-ceo-says-56000-annually-for-alzheimers-drug-is-fair-promises-not-to-hike-price-for-at-least-4-years.html#:~:text=Health%20and%20Science-,Biogen%20CEO%20says%20%2456%2C000%20annually%20for%20Alzheimer's%20drug%20is%20'fair,for%20at%20least%204%20years&text=Biogen%20CEO%20Michel%20Vounatsos%20told,drug%20aducanumab%20is%20%E2%80%9Cfair.%E2%80%9D
[96] https://www.sciencehistory.org/distillations/frontline-pharmacies
[97] ibid
[98] Clin Infect Dis. 1993 Apr;16(4):580-4. doi: 10.1093/clind/16.4.580., https://pubmed.ncbi.nlm.nih.gov/8513069/
[99] https://www.wellrx.com/news/the-history-of-american-pharmacies/
[100] Home > Committees > House Oversight and Reform
[101] ibid
[102] https://www.statnews.com/2015/12/11/untold-story-tvs-first-prescription-drug-ad/
[103] https://www.rasmussen.edu/degrees/health-sciences/blog/types-of-pharmacies/
[104] https://www.indeed.com/hire/job-description/pharmacy-technician?gclid=Cj0KCQjw6NmHBhD2ARIsAI3hrM0cwgmF3LnqIJQfqMOaNEhxaj6e0rKtTF0Zv8hM-X77K-29O2m0VzsaAmCFEALw_wcB&aceid=
[105] https://www.indeed.com/career/pharmacy-technician/salaries/CA
[106] Further clarification is found in the California Legislative SB 1039: A pharmacy with only one pharmacist shall have no more than one pharmacy technician performing the tasks specified in subdivision (a). The ratio of pharmacy technicians performing the tasks specified in subdivision (a) to any additional pharmacist shall not exceed 2:1, except that this ratio shall not apply to personnel performing clerical functions pursuant to Section 4116 or 4117. This ratio is applicable to all practice settings, except for an inpatient of a licensed health facility, a patient of a licensed home health agency, as specified in paragraph (2), an inmate of a correctional facility of the Department of

Corrections and Rehabilitation, and for a person receiving treatment in a facility operated by the State Department of State Hospitals, the State Department of Developmental Services, or the Department of Veterans Affairs.

[107] Malacos, Kristy. "Pharmacy Technician Regulation." Pharmacy Times. Pharmacy & Healthcare Communications, LLC. Retrieved 1 July 2018.

[108] https://www.ncbi.nlm.nih.gov/pmc/articles/PMC5155458/

[109] https://cvshealth.com/about-cvs-health/our-purpose/our-history

[110]https://www.google.com/search?q=what+is+cvs+annual+revenue&sxsrf=ALeKk02hm4K7c6TSrMgodj9DfmuAgs6xiQ%3A1626298768150&ei=kFnvYOrECNC-0PEP1YCL0A8&oq=what+is+cvs+revenue&gs_lcp=Cgdnd3Mtd2l6EAEYADIGCAAQFhAeMgUIABCGAzIFCAAQhgM6BQgAEJECOggIABCxAxCDAToLCC4QsQMQxwEQowI6DgguELEDEIMBEMcBEKMCOgUIABCxAzoICC4QxwEQowI6BAgjECc6BAgAEEM6AggAOgUIABDJAzoFCAAQkgM6CAgAEMkDEJECOgQIABAKSgQIQRgAUPmJ9wFYtsb3AWDb5PcBaABwAngAgAHMAYgBixSSAQYxLjE4LjGYAQCgAQGqAQdnd3Mtd2l6wAEB&sclient=gws-wiz

[111] Ellen Gabler, The New York Times, FEB 03, 2020, https://www.chicagotribune.com/business/ct-biz-nyt-pharmacy-mistakes-20200201-wp2ftrt2sjhfvjwnmwbtnl3y3i-story.html

[112] https://www.drugtopics.com/view/independent-pharmacies-not-dead-yet

[113] Richard Adams Blog, The Guardian, Wed 21 Apr 2010

[114] Medscape Internist Compensation Report 2020, Keith L. Martin, May 20, 2020

[115] Ibid, page 9

[116] Ibid, page 3

[117] Ibid, page 20

[118] Ibid, page 17

[119] Trends in Healthcare Spending, August 13, 2019, Copyright 1995 - 2020 American Medical Association. All rights reserved.

[120] NORC at the University of Chicago https://www.norc.org/Research/Projects/Pages/WHI-NORC-Aging-Survey.aspx

[121] CMS, Centers for Medicare and Medicaid Services

[122] ICD-1 to ICD-11 Timeline Highlights Healthcare's Evolution, By Jacqueline DiChiara, August 11, 2015, RevCycleIntelligence, published by Xtelligent Healthcare Media, LLC.

[123] Statista, Health Care, The U.S. Has the Most Expensive Healthcare System in the World, by
Niall McCarthy, https://www.statista.com/chart/8658/health-spending-per-capita/#:~:text=The%20U.S.%20Has%20the%20Most%20Expensive%20Healthcare%20System%20in%20the%20World,-by%20Niall%20McCarthy, Aug 8, 2019
[124] ibid
[125] © 2020 Blue Cross Blue Shield Association. All Rights Reserved.
[126] © 2020 Kaiser Foundation Health Plan, Inc., https://healthy.kaiserpermanente.org/shop-plans/which-plan-is-for-me
[127] Kaiser Health news, Accountable Care Organizations, Explained, By Jenny Gold, September 14, 2015
[128] Kaiser Health News with support from The SCAN Foundation, Jenny Gold: jgold@kff.org, @JennyAGold
[129] Medscape Internist Compensation Report 2020, Keith L. Martin, page 20
[130] Copyright WordHippo © 2020
[131] University of California, Berkeley, People and Culture, Copyright © 2020 UC Regents; all rights reserved
[132] AAPA Guidelines for Ethical Conduct for the PA Professional, https://www.aapa.org/wp-content/uploads/2017/02/16-EthicalConduct.pdf
[133] American Association of Nurse Practitioners, Standards of Practice, https://www.aanp.org/advocacy/advocacy-resource/position-statements/standards-of-practice-for-nurse-practitioners
[134] Understanding the Fundamentals of Accountable Care Organizations, ©2012-2020 Xtelligent Healthcare Media, LLC. All rights reserved. RevCycleIntelligence.com is published by Xtelligent Healthcare Media, LLC Apr 5, 2019
[135] Wall Street Journal, "Doctors, Once GOP Stalwarts, Now More Likely to Be Democrats," By Janet Adamy and Paul Overberg, Oct. 6, 2019
[136] The Hidden System that Explains How Your Doctor Makes Referrals, WSJ, By Anna Wilde Mathews and Melanie Evans, Dec. 27, 2018
[137] Ibid
[138] Special Health Care for Congress: Lawmakers' Health Care Perks, Jay Shaylor and Mark Abdelmalek, Sept. 30, 2009
[139] Fang X (2012). Barefoot doctors and western medicine in China.

ISBN 9781580464338. OCLC 779874566
[140] Gong, Y. L.; Chao, L. M. (September 1982). "The role of barefoot doctors." American Journal of Public Health. 72 (9 Suppl): 59–61.
[141] Dong Z, Phillips MR (November 2008). "Evolution of China's health-care system." Lancet. 372
[142] Fang X (2012). Barefoot doctors and western medicine in China.
[143] "Health Information - Beijing, China - Embassy of the United States." usembassy-china.org.cn. Archived from the original
[144] Resources: https://en.wikipedia.org/wiki/Healthcare_in_China
[145] Traditional and Modern Chinese Medicine, https://en.wikipedia.org/wiki/Healthcare_in_China
[146] Li X, Chongsuvivatwong V, Xia X, Sangsupawanich P, Zheng W, Ma K (August 2012). "Revisiting current "barefoot doctors" in border areas of China: system of services, financial issue and clinical practice prior to introducing integrated management of childhood illness (IMCI)"
[147] https://en.wikipedia.org/wiki/Healthcare_in_China
[148] http://news.xinhuanet.com/english/2016-02/26/c_135131604.htm
[149] Quality of primary health care in China: challenges and recommendations, Xi Li, PhD, Prof Harlan M Krumholz, MD, Prof Winnie Yip, PhD, Prof Kar Keung Cheng, FMedSci, Prof Jan De Maeseneer, PhD, Prof Qingyue Meng, PhD, Published: June 06, 2020, DOI:https://doi.org/10.1016/S0140-6736(20)30122-7
[150] "Scalped: At China's creaking hospitals, illegal ticket touts defy crackdown." Reuters. 12 April 2016. Retrieved 13 April 2016.
[151] ibid
[152] Final Diagnosis, ©Roger C. Dunham, 1993, Penguin Press, L.A. County Hospital Jail Ward
[153]March 2000,Journal of Burn Care & Rehabilitation 21(2):112-4, Craig E. Amshel, Daniel M. Caruso
[154] Estimated Influenza Illnesses, Medical visits, Hospitalizations, and death, www.cdc.gov Jan 8, 2020
[155] Travel China Guide: https://www.travelchinaguide.com/
[156] Steven Novella (25 January 2012). "What Is Traditional Chinese Medicine?" Archived from the original on 15 April 2014
[157] Medieval European medicine and Asian spices, PubMedpubmed.ncbi.nlm.nih.gov
[158] Huangdi Neijing, Wikipedia, https://en.wikipedia.org/wiki/Huangdi_Neijing
[159] © UNHCR 2020, https://www.unhcr.org/ China: Whether medical doctors in China swear the Hippocratic oath or an equivalent

[160] China - Chinadaily.com.cnwww.chinadaily.com.cn, Apr 21, 2017
[161] Chinese patient testimonial
[162] Personal commentary from Chinese citizen
[163] The Borgen Project, Stefanie Grodman, https://borgenproject.org/homelessness-in-china/
[164] ibid
[165] History of Western Medicine in China, Resources Portal, Med Hist. 2016 Oct; 60(4): 609–610, Reviewed by David Luesink
[166] Popovich, L (2011). "Russian Federation: Health system review" (PDF). Health Systems in Transition. 13 (7): 1–190
[167] Density of doctors in Russia 2010-2018, Published by D. Elagina, Jun 17, 2020
[168] A Census of Actively Licensed Physicians in the United States, 2016, Aaron Young, PhD; Humayun J. Chaudhry, DO, MS; Xiaomei Pei, PhD; Katie Arnhart, PhD; Michael Dugan, MBA; and Gregory B. Snyder, MD
[169] Britnell, Mark (2015). In Search of the Perfect Health System. London: Palgrave. pp. 81–84
[170] Expatica, July 27, 2020, © 2000 - 2020
[171] https://en.bookimed.com/create-order/select-procedure-illness?clinicId=371&type=messenger-priority&questionTag=skype&doctorId=1372&button=listing-doctor-btn
[172] https://en.wikipedia.org/wiki/List_of_Russian_physicians_and_psychologists
[173] Royal Museums Greenwich, Health in the 17th Century, https://www.rmg.co.uk/stories/topics/health-17th-century
[174] By the editors of the Encyclopedia Britannica, https://www.britannica.com/science/leeching
[175] PBS, https://www.pbs.org/newshour/show/bloodletting-blisters-solving-medical-mystery-george-washingtons-death
[176] The Fred W. Smith National Library for George Washington, The Death of George Washington, https://www.mountvernon.org/library/digitalhistory/digital-encyclopedia/article/the-death-of-george-washington/?gclid=CjwKCAjw3riIBhAwEiwAzD3TiVjmhKbbPfCc6QTDBLOkQlWEXFfPvkf7LNGVCSkU82Og0PwuNxlKkRoCAAEQAvD_BwE
[177] Wikipedia, https://en.wikipedia.org/wiki/Royal_touch
[178] Wikipedia, List of Medical Schools in the United Kingdom, https://en.wikipedia.org/wiki/List_of_medical_schools_in_the_United

_Kingdom
[179] Rossi, Ann (2006). Two Cultures Meet: Native American and European. National Geographic Society. pp. 31–32. ISBN 978-0792286790.
[180] Hanna, Charles A.: The wilderness trail : or, the ventures and adventures of the Pennsylvania traders on the Allegheny path, with some new annals of the old West, and the records of some strong men and some bad ones (1911) pg.366
[181] For Burning with Gunnpowder or otherwise. Stafford, Ed. (Edward), 1617-. Receipts to cure various disorders for my worthy friend Mr. Winthrop, by Edward Stafford, 1643 May 6. B MS b76, Countway Library of Medicine
[182] My Black powder against ye plague, small pox, purples, all sorts of feavers; Poyson; either by Way of prevention, or after Infection. Edward Stafford, 1643
[183] Tufts, Cotton, 1732-1815. Receipt book of Cotton Tufts, 1773-1784 (inclusive). B MS b11.1, Countway Library of Medicine.
[184] Harvard University Cambridge, MA, "Medicine in Colonial North America" Essay by 2016 Arcadia Fellow Theresa McCulla
[185] Ibid
[186] ibid
[187] The UK health care system, By Lee Tunstall, Prepared for EvidenceNetwork.ca
[188] ibid
[189] ibid
[190] Swearing to care: the resurgence in medical oaths, Hurwitz B, Richardson R, BMJ. 1997 Dec 20-27; 315(7123):1671-4.
[191] Personal Communication with London residents
[192] ActiveQuote, What does Private Health Insurance cost? By David Woodfield 3rd October 2018
[193] Roosa Tikkanen, Robin Osborn, Elias Mossialos, Ana Djordjevic, and George A. Wharton, June 5, 2020, https://www.commonwealthfund.org/international-health-policy-center/countries/england
[194] ibid
[195]HomeUtility Navigation NEWSROOM TO THE POINT, Affordable, quality health care, HEALTH AND SYSTEM STATISTICS England, June 5, 2020, Roosa Tikkanen, Robin Osborn, Elias Mossialos, Ana Djordjevic, and George A. Wharton
[196] Institute for Fiscal Studies (IFS), The characteristics and incomes of

the top 1%, Robert Joyce, Thomas Pope and Barra Roantree, Briefing note, 06 Aug 2019

[197] Malcolm G. Taylor. The Seven Decisions That Created the Canadian Health Insurance System and Their Outcomes. Second edition. McGill-Queen's University Press, 1987.

[198] The Lancet, Canada's Universal Health-care System: Achieving Its Potential, February 22, 2018

[199] Department of Justice, Canada, Canada Health Act, CHAPTER C-6, https://web.archive.org/web/20031206135446/http://laws.justice.gc.ca/en/C-6/15944.html#rid-16009

[200] https://en.wikipedia.org/wiki/Canada_Health_Act

[201] Violations and Penalties, https://en.wikipedia.org/wiki/Canada_Health_Act

[202] Reports and Publications - Canada Health Act Annual Reports, Government of Canada, https://www.canada.ca/en/health-canada/services/health-care-system/reports-publications/canada-health-act-annual-reports.html

[203] Personal report, Val Muth, province of Ontario

[204] Fraser Institute, https://www.fraserinstitute.org/article/canadas-doctor-shortage-will-only-worsen-in-the-coming-decade

[205] ibid

[206] Reuters World News, July 12, 2020, Foreign Doctors' Hopes for Fast-Track Pandemic Licenses in Canada Fading, By Moira Warburton

[207] Organization for Economic Co-operation and Development, currently the following countries: They are Austria, Belgium, Czech Republic, Denmark, Estonia, Finland, France, Germany, Greece, Hungary, Iceland, Ireland, Italy, Latvia, Lithuania, Luxembourg, Netherlands, Norway, Poland, Portugal, Slovak Republic, Slovenia, Spain, Sweden, Switzerland, and the United Kingdom.

[208] ibid

[209] Stastica, https://www.statista.com/statistics/831118/canada-family-general-practitioners-by-province/

[210] The Canadian Encyclopedia, Medical Ethics, by Patricia G. Bailey and Benjamin Freedman, Published Online, Last Edited, July 7, 2015

[211] Royal College of Physicians and Surgeons in Canada, "Medical Ethics: Past, Present and Future,"
Heather MacDougall, PhD, Associate Professor, Department of History, University of Waterloo, G. Ross Langley MD, FRCPC, MACP, FRCP, Emeritus Professor of Medicine, Dalhousie University

[212] ibid

[213] ibid
[214] Canadian Medical Association Code of Ethics and Professionalism, https://policybase.cma.ca/documents/policypdf/PD19-03.pdf
[215] Medical School Admission Statistics, https://mededits.com/medical-school-admissions/statistics/
[216] ibid
[217] Rely MD, https://relymd.com/blog-infographic-average-wait-times-to-see-a-doctor/#:~:text=For%20primary%20care%20physicians%2C%20patients,same%20day%20they%20need%20care.
[218] Physician Assistants and Their Role in Primary Care, James F. Cawley, MPH, PA-C, https://journalofethics.ama-assn.org/article/physician-assistants-and-their-role-primary-care/2012-05
[219] CMS Statistics booklet, https://www.cms.gov/Research-Statistics-Data-and-Systems/Statistics-Trends-and-Reports/CMS-Statistics-Reference-Booklet/Downloads/CMS_Stats_2010.pdf
[220] Healthcare Dive, Published January 28, 2019, Les Masterson
[221] https://www.kff.org/other/state-indicator/total-medical-school-graduates/?currentTimeframe=0&selectedRows=%7B%22states%22:%7B%22california%22:%7B%7D%7D%7D&sortModel=%7B%22colId%22:%22Location%22,%22sort%22:%22asc%22%7D
[222] New Findings Confirm Predictions on Physician Shortage, APRIL 23, 2019, https://www.aamc.org/news-insights/press-releases/new-findings-confirm-predictions-physician-shortage
[223] Current Procedural Terminology (CPT) code, Margaret Rouse, https://searchhealthit.techtarget.com/definition/Current-Procedural-Terminology-CPT#:~:text=Current%20Procedural%20Terminology%20(CPT)%20is,insurance%20companies%20and%20accreditation%20organizations.&text=CPT%20is%20a%20registered%20trademark%20of%20the%20American%20Medical%20Association
[224] Forbes, Why the American Medical Association Had 72 Million Reasons to Shrink Doctors' Pay, The Apothecary, Avik Roy, Forbes, https://www.forbes.com/sites/theapothecary/2011/11/28/why-the-american-medical-association-had-72-million-reasons-to-help-shrink-doctors-pay/?sh=7e0d60a460d9
The ApothecaryContributor Group
Policy
[225] AMA: Employed physicians outnumber self-employed, May 6, 2019,

https://www.ama-assn.org/press-center/press-releases/employed-physicians-outnumber-self-employed

[226] ibid

[227] Healthcare Weekly, December 20, 2018, "29 percent of U.S. doctors are born outside the U.S., new study shows," Anca Spanu, American Healthcare System, Immigrants, U.S. Doctors Study

[228] Health, December 4, 2018, U.S. relies heavily on foreign-born healthcare workers, By Lisa Rapaport, Reuters Health

[229] American Immigration Council, "Foreign-Trained Doctors are Critical to Serving Many U.S. Communities," Special Report, January, 2018, www.AmericanImmigrationCouncil.org, and www.ImmigrationImpact.com

[230] Seattle Magazine, Why Concierge Care is Becoming More Popular in Seattle, by Malia Jacobson, February, 2016

[231] https://www.virginiamason.org/concierge-medicine

[232] Owler, MDVIP's Competitors, Revenue, Number of Employees, Funding, Acquisitions & News, https://www.owler.com/company/mdvip

[233] Modern Healthcare, February 18, 2015, Concierge physicians rattled by $8.5 million liability award, Andis Robeznieks

[234] MDVIP, "For Patients," https://www.mdvip.com/patients/frequently-asked-questions

[235] MDVIP, https://www.mdvip.com/patients/frequently-asked-questions

[236] Owler, MDVIP's Competitors, Revenue, Number of Employees, Funding, Acquisitions & News, https://www.owler.com/company/mdvip

Made in the USA
Las Vegas, NV
04 March 2026

43064753R00223